The Complete GPVTS Stage 2 Preparation Guide

Questions and Professional Dilemmas

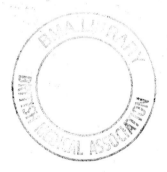

The Complete GPVTS Stage 2 Preparation Guide

Questions and Professional Dilemmas

Edited by

Saba Khan MBBS, DFFP, DRCOG, MRCGP
(Distinction), MSc
GP and Programme Director, Chertsey GPVTS, KSS
Deanery

with **Neel Sharma** BSc (Hons), MBChB, MSc
Core Medical Trainee Year One, Lewisham Healthcare
NHS Trust and Honorary Clinical Lecturer in Medical
Education, Barts and the London School of Medicine
and Dentistry

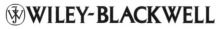

WILEY-BLACKWELL

A John Wiley & Sons, Ltd., Publication

This edition first published 2012 © 2012 by John Wiley & Sons, Ltd.

Wiley-Blackwell is an imprint of John Wiley & Sons, formed by the merger of Wiley's global Scientific, Technical and Medical business with Blackwell Publishing.

Registered Office
John Wiley & Sons, Ltd, The Atrium, Southern Gate, Chichester, West Sussex, PO19 8SQ, UK

Editorial Offices
9600 Garsington Road, Oxford, OX4 2DQ, UK
The Atrium, Southern Gate, Chichester, West Sussex, PO19 8SQ, UK
111 River Street, Hoboken, NJ 07030-5774, USA

For details of our global editorial offices, for customer services and for information about how to apply for permission to reuse the copyright material in this book please see our website at www.wiley.com/wiley-blackwell.

The right of the author to be identified as the author of this work has been asserted in accordance with the UK Copyright, Designs and Patents Act 1988.

Library of Congress Cataloging-in-Publication Data

Khan, Saba.
The complete GPVTS stage 2 preparation guide : questions and professional dilemmas / edited by Saba Khan with Neel Sharma.
    p. ; cm.
  Includes bibliographical references and index.
  ISBN-13: 978-0-470-65490-3 (pbk. : alk. paper)
  ISBN-10: 0-470-65490-2 (pbk. : alk. paper)
I. Sharma, Neel. II. Title.
[DNLM: 1. General Practice–education–Great Britain–Examination Questions.
2. General Practitioners–education–Great Britain–Examination Questions. WB 18.2]
  LC classification not assigned
  610.76–dc23

                    2011029725

A catalogue record for this book is available from the British Library.

This book is published in the following electronic formats: ePDF 9781119959854; ePub 9781119959861; Mobi 9781119959878

Set in 9.25/11.5pt Minion by SPi Publisher Services, Pondicherry, India
Printed and bound in Malaysia by Vivar Printing Sdn Bhd

1   2012

Contents

Contributors

Safia Debar
MSc, MBBS, DCH, DRCOG, nMRCGP, DipOccMed
GP, NIHR In-practice Fellow

Ounali Jaffer
FRCR, MRCP, MBBS
Radiologist
Kings College Hospital London

Neman S Khan
MRCGP, DFFP, DRCOG, MBBS
GP Principle and Trainer, Working

Saba Khan
MBBS, DFFP, DRCOG, MRCGP (Distinction), MSc
GP and Programme Director, Chertsey GPVTS, KSS Deanery

Donna Pilkington
BSc, MBChB
GPST1 Trainee

Neel Sharma
BSc (Hons), MBChB, MSc
Core Medical Trainee Year One, Lewisham Healthcare NHS Trust
and Honorary Clinical Lecturer in Medical Education,
Barts and the London School of Medicine and Dentistry

The Complete GPVTS Stage 2 Preparation Guide

This book has been written with the aspiring GP in mind, and it should contain enough information for you to be able to feel confident about taking and passing the Stage 2 entrance exam.

The entrance process is made up of four parts. This book is a guide for the second part of this process and should help you gain enough practice to feel more able to pass this stage comfortably.

Stage 1

The first stage is essentially completion of your application form, and producing evidence that you have completed training competently to then be able to apply for further specialty training.

The National Person Specification is a document that outlines all of the qualifications and attributes necessary to apply successfully for GP specialty training. It is worth being aware of the GMC Good Medical Practice guide as eligibility is based on these seven criteria. There are also six criteria under the Personal Skills section that are worth reading through that should be covered within your answers on the application form. The person specification also covers health and probity. There are standardised pieces of evidence that need to be provided at this stage of the process and details of this are on the National Recruitment Office (NRO) website (www.gprecruitment.org.uk).

As an applicant in this process you also need to clearly show evidence of having reached Foundation Competency through approved training posts. Those applicants who have come from other specialties or who have had gaps in training will need to present evidence of competency in line with GMC Standards.

The application form is submitted online, and once completed cannot be altered unless there are very specific reasons for a change to your preferred choice of deanery. When applying it is important to look at the geographical areas covered by each deanery, as your ranking of four preferred deanery choices will influence where you are offered a place.

Stage 2

The second stage is a computer-based assessment that will determine shortlisting and allocation for Stage 3 of the selection process. Candidates will complete this computer-based exam at various Pearson Vue centres around the UK. The Pearson Vue website can be used to book the test and also as a resource for a practical tutorial on how to record your answers on the day.

The paper is made up of two parts: a Professional Dilemma section followed by a Clinical Problem Solving section.

From previous papers, it is best to allow at least two hours for the Professional Dilemma and approximately one hour for the Clinical Problem Solving.

The Professional Dilemma section contains two types of question. The first is a ranking question, where the candidate is given a scenario and asked to rank the five options in order of most suitable response down to least appropriate. This is an exercise in decision making and rationalisation.

The second type of question sets out a scenario and asks the candidate to typically select three options from a list of answers, in any order, as their management plan or best response.

These questions are not negatively marked and in fact have a 'most right answer' which is judged as the best possible response for a competent doctor at F2 level. If the candidate selects a different but still reasonable response, marks will still be awarded. It is therefore advisable to attempt all questions as there are marks available even if the ideal answer is not chosen.

The second part of the assessment is made up of the Clinical Problem Solving section. This exam tests your ability to apply your clinical knowledge to various clinical scenarios. It does not expect a working knowledge of general practice but rather a competent approach and knowledge level appropriate to a foundation stage doctor, regardless of the patient presentation.

The answer totals are collated into four bands which are based on a range of scores, so those with the highest scores fall into the highest band and those with the lowest scores fall into the lowest band. The scores that trainees attain in this assessment will influence the allocation of their preferred deanery post, because the deaneries with higher demand for training posts will award rotations to candidates with higher scores first. Unfortunately those trainees that fall into the lowest band are not shortlisted.

Scoring for previous exams can be accessed on the NRO website.

Stage 3

The results from Stage 2 are used to allocate and rank candidates to their preferred deanery. The candidates are then assigned to a selection centre for Stage 3 assessment. The deanery assigned to each candidate will be more likely to be their first choice, the higher their score in the second stage. Those candidates with lower scores will be given their second choice and so on, dependent on available places. If none of the four choices can be met, vacant rotations in any deanery could be offered.

The Stage 3 assessment requires three references from recent educational and clinical supervisors, which should be recorded on the structured reference forms available on the NRO website. Along with these references a number of personal documents will also be required.

The Stage 3 assessment consists of two components: a simulation exercise and a written exercise.

The simulation exercise is made up of three 10-minute scenarios, designed to test the main attributes outlined in the National Person Specification.

The 10-minute scenarios are with a simulator who will act the part of a relative/carer, a patient and also a non-medical colleague. The role play is designed to test skills such as communication, empathy and problem solving. Clinical skills or knowledge are not tested in this process as it is the more difficult skills of patient and doctor interaction that are being assessed.

The written exercise will last approximately 30 minutes and will require the candidate to prioritise and justify their response to a dilemma presented to them. This exercise, again, is not designed to test clinical knowledge but to assess decision-making skills.

This part of the assessment is more focused on professionalism and rationalisation, hence it is best to try and use best judgement and common sense rather than relying on textbook answers.

Stage 4

Stage 4 of the assessment process involves the collation of results from Stage 2 and Stage 3. Once these results are collated all candidates are ranked in order, and those with the highest ranking are offered their first choice of deanery. Candidates are then offered their remaining choices of deanery if their first choice is unavailable. Following this, those candidates who are not given an offer may be offered a place in a different deanery to those on their preferred list, through local and then national clearing.

How to Use This Book

This book is designed to help you tease out where your strengths and possible learning gaps are. It is a useful aid at the beginning of your exam preparation to help guide learning or toward the end of your revision to make sure that you have all areas covered.

In our experience exam preparation is a balance between how much you know and how much you can apply what you know. The questions in this book are designed to test how much you know and the explanations will help you to test whether you are applying this knowledge correctly.

One of the most challenging aspects to the Stage 2 exam is the time pressure, which in itself is a key skill to becoming a good General Practitioner. The papers are written to test how you work under pressure as opposed to making subject matter unfairly difficult. Much of the skill of developing as a generalist lies in your ability to negotiate a large amount of work in a relatively small amount of time. This is an essential skill that is worth paying attention to prior to this process.

It would be helpful to use different chapters under timed conditions to see how you cope with this aspect of the exam.

The exam is designed to test Foundation level knowledge and does not expect you to have a working knowledge of General Practice. However the topics that you come across in the questions are commonly seen in General Practice. Much of your knowledge will come from learning that you have already done during your clinical posts as well as more structured teaching opportunities that you may have had. To support this we recommend standard clinical texts that cover general medicine, surgery and the specialties. However, this should be selective learning, based on where you find your learning needs are, after covering some of the subject matter in this book.

The chapters have been divided by subject to help you find where you need to focus your learning, with explanations to aid this. We have used authors with both experience and expertise in each subject area to make the questions as fair as possible.

The Professional Dilemma section is not a knowledge-based exercise. The scenarios are designed to assess the candidate's ability to make clear and sound judgements, in difficult ethical or professional situations. These are real issues that could easily arise in one's own practice. For revision purposes, a useful resource is the GMC's *Good Medical Practice Guide*.

It is worth spending time looking over this document to be aware of the domains that could be covered.

The questions are written with options with a most correct answer moving down to a least correct answer, there are still marks awarded if answers are not in the key response order but are almost correct. In these scenarios it is best to use standards such as the GMC guidance as your best plan of action.

Exam Technique

The Professional Dilemma paper for 2010 contained 60 questions, which were made up of ranking 4–5 options or selecting 2–3 responses for an answer stem. We recommend that for the ranking questions it is best to put the most suitable answer first, the least suitable answer last, and then arrange the remaining responses. These questions are more focused on your ability as a practitioner to sensibly deal with more difficult scenarios commonly faced by medical professionals. These questions are not designed to trip you up or to be difficult, they are purely a test of your decision-making ability. This is something that all clinicians do on a day-to-day basis regardless of their specialty field. However, in General Practice it is done at a much faster rate and under very specific time limits and this skill is tested in this paper.

It is good exam technique to try and answer as many questions as possible as each question has equal weighting; rather than spending too long on a few questions it is best to answer as many as possible. This is the main difficulty of this paper and we recommend working on the dilemma section of this book under timed conditions to help you develop this skill.

There is no negative marking in this paper so reasonable attempts at all questions should be made.

For the Clinical Problem Solving paper, there were 105 questions. The majority of the questions are based on general medicine with a smaller proportion allocated to the specialties. With the use of this book, you can focus your learning into areas where you may have more knowledge gaps, and focus your revision into these areas. However this exam is not designed to be difficult but is specifically aimed at Foundation level competency.

One of the most challenging aspects to this exam is the time pressure involved in the completion of each paper. It is worth attempting questions under timed conditions for this section also, to assess your own ability in this area.

We also recommend picking questions that you know you can answer quickly and then moving to the ones that are more difficult for you to do later in the exam. However, this requires you to look through the paper before starting, and some candidates would prefer to just start working and push through in order not to waste time. It is worth looking at which technique works for you and how you work best.

The Stage 3 assessment is much more about professionalism, and requires each candidate to demonstrate good judgement in an empathic and clear way. It is worth spending some time looking through the GMC website, as there are some excellent learning resources that will help focus your learning. The National Person Specification is also important for this part of your revision as much of this entire process is based on these principles. It is also helpful to practise different scenarios with colleagues to help you develop your skills.

Again, this stage is about how you demonstrate your professionalism in a pressurised situation. The examiners will be looking for candidates to remain focused and to give clear, considered judgements. The decisions expected to be made by each candidate are those that should fall within the realms of what is considered safe and reasonable for doctors at Foundation level competency. It is best to be natural and make sure you can justify the decisions that you make.

In summary, this exam is designed to ensure that those opting for General Practice are suited to the process and possess the necessary qualities to progress through training.

This book will, it is hoped, help guide your revision and ensure that you have a successful outcome!

Part 1

Clinical Problem Solving Questions: SBAs and EMQs

1 Cardiology

Single best answer questions

For each question below, what is the most likely answer?
Select ONE option only from the answers supplied.

1. A 76-year-old man presents to his GP. He complains of breathlessness
   which is made worse on exertion. He denies any history of chest pain or
   a cough. He has a past medical history of asthma which was diagnosed
   as a child. On examination you note a blood pressure of 123/77 mmHg,
   pulse rate of 67 beats per minute and a temperature of 36.7°C.
   Cardiovascular examination reveals a low-pitched diastolic murmur
   over the apex. Respiratory examination proves unremarkable. What is
   the most likely diagnosis?
   a) Mitral regurgitation
   b) Aortic stenosis
   c) Pulmonary stenosis
   d) Mitral stenosis
   e) Aortic regurgitation

2. A 52-year-old Bengali man is referred to the cardiology outpatient
   department by his GP due to concerns with his blood pressure. A blood
   pressure diary reveals readings over 160/100 mmHg over a 2-week
   period. Fundoscopy examination proves unremarkable. What is the
   most suitable management option?
   a) Watch and wait
   b) Repeat blood pressure measurement in one week
   c) Commence amlodipine
   d) Commence ramipril
   e) Commence bendroflumethiazide

3. A 79-year-old woman presents to the Emergency Department. She
   complains of central chest pain which came on at rest. Background
   medical history includes type 2 diabetes and hypercholesterolaemia.

The Complete GPVTS Stage 2 Preparation Guide: Questions and Professional Dilemmas,
First Edition. Edited by Saba Khan with Neel Sharma.
© 2012 John Wiley & Sons, Ltd. Published 2012 by John Wiley & Sons, Ltd.

You note that she is quite short of breath with a pulse rate of 115 beats per minute and blood pressure of 95/45 mmHg. What is the single most important investigation in this case?

a) ECHO
b) ECG
c) Chest X-ray
d) Serum troponin
e) Arterial blood gas

4. A 46-year-old man attends the Emergency Department. He complains of central chest pain which is worse on inspiration. An ECG demonstrates evidence of diffuse concave ST elevation. What is the most likely diagnosis?

a) Myocardial infarction
b) Costochondritis
c) Pericarditis
d) Pulmonary embolism
e) Gastro-oesophageal reflux disease

5. A 23-year-old male hockey player collapses suddenly during a match and is rushed to the Emergency Department. He is noted to be in asystole on arrival and despite the best efforts of the resuscitation doctors is pronounced dead. No trauma was sustained during the match. What is the most likely cause of death?

a) Hypertrophic cardiomyopathy
b) Myocardial infarction
c) Pulmonary embolism
d) Aortic dissection
e) Commotio cordis

6. A 42-year-old man presents to the Emergency Department. He complains of left-sided chest discomfort and generalised weakness. He has a background history of hypertension and type 2 diabetes. An ECG demonstrates evidence of a shortened PR interval and a slow rise of the initial upstroke of the QRS complex. What is the most likely diagnosis?

a) Hypertrophic cardiomyopathy
b) Vasovagal syncope
c) First-degree heart block
d) Atrial fibrillation
e) Wolff-Parkinson-White syndrome

7. Which of the following is NOT a contraindication to exercise stress testing?

a) Left main coronary artery stenosis
b) Severe mitral regurgitation
c) Aortic dissection
d) Severe aortic stenosis
e) Severe osteoarthritis

8. You are the F2 doctor on call and are asked to see a 63-year-old woman. On arrival the nurse informs you that the patient has a strong cardiac history. An ECG demonstrates a narrow QRS complex and a regular rhythm. Which of the following is the most appropriate initial treatment?
   a) Adenosine
   b) Atropine
   c) DC cardioversion
   d) Adrenaline
   e) Amiodarone

9. An 82-year-old woman presents to the Emergency Department. Routine observations reveal a blood pressure of 85/45 mmHg and pulse rate of 162 beats per minute. Which of the following is the most appropriate initial treatment?
   a) Valsalva manoeuvre
   b) Adenosine
   c) Amiodarone
   d) DC cardioversion
   e) Bisoprolol

10. A 69-year-old man is reviewed by his GP. He complains of chest pain which is worse on inspiration, as well as a fever. He has recently been discharged from hospital following a myocardial infarction 7 weeks prior. On examination you note a pulse rate of 72 beats per minute and blood pressure of 124/75 mmHg. Cardiovascular examination reveals evidence of a rub over the left lower sternal edge. What is the most likely diagnosis?
    a) Dressler's syndrome
    b) Pneumonia
    c) Pulmonary embolism
    d) Cardiac tamponade
    e) Pericarditis

11. A 63-year-old woman is admitted to hospital with central chest pain, radiating to her left arm. She has a background history of hypertension. On examination her heart sounds are normal with no audible murmurs. Routine observations demonstrate a pulse rate of 96 beats per minute and blood pressure of 142/93 mmHg. An ECG demonstrates evidence of ST depression. Which one of the following is the most suitable initial management?
    a) Aspirin 75 mg
    b) Aspirin 75 mg and clopidogrel 75 mg
    c) Bisoprolol 5 mg
    d) Aspirin 300 mg, clopidogrel 300 mg, enoxaparin 1 mg/kg
    e) Aspirin 300 mg, clopidogrel 300 mg, enoxaparin 1 mg/kg and bisoprolol 5 mg

12. A 45-year-old man is admitted to the Emergency Department. He complains of a 2-hour history of sudden-onset central crushing chest pain. An ECG demonstrates evidence of ST elevation in anterior leads. Which of the following is the most suitable management option?
    a) Aspirin 75 mg
    b) Clopidogrel 75 mg
    c) Dobutamine stress echo
    d) Exercise treadmill test
    e) Coronary angiography

13. A 78-year-old woman is reviewed by her GP for a routine check-up. She has a strong cardiac history and required some urgent blood tests. Results demonstrate a serum sodium of 128 mmol/L, a potassium of 5.9 mmol/L, urea of 3.2 mmol/L and a creatinine of 88 μmol/L. Which of the following drugs is the most likely cause for her blood results?
    a) Spironolactone
    b) Bumetanide
    c) Furosemide
    d) Bendroflumethiazide
    e) Atenolol

14. A 28-year-old woman presents to her GP following an episode of syncope. She has a background history of schizophrenia which was recently diagnosed. She was commenced on risperidone orally and has been compliant with her medication. Full system examination proves unremarkable. What is the most likely diagnosis?
    a) Vasovagal syncope
    b) Postural hypotension
    c) Hypertrophic cardiomyopathy
    d) Sick sinus syndrome
    e) Long QT syndrome

15. A 54-year-old woman presents to her GP. She complains of generalised abdominal discomfort over a 2-week period. On examination you note evidence of a white discoloration of her retina and hepatosplenomegaly. What is the most likely diagnosis?
    a) Type I hyperlipoproteinaemia
    b) Type II hyperlipoproteinaemia
    c) Type III hyperlipoproteinaemia
    d) Type IV hyperlipoproteinaemia
    e) Type V hyperlipoproteinaemia

Extended matching questions

Question 1
a) Furosemide
b) Atenolol
c) Ramipril
d) Spironolactone
e) Amlodipine
f) Bendroflumethiazide
g) Bisoprolol
h) Amiodarone

For each patient below, what is the most likely cause?
Select ONE option only from the list above.
Each option may be selected once, more than once or not at all.

1. A 62-year-old woman with a background history of hypertension and increased ankle swelling.
2. A 78-year-old man presenting with shortness of breath and visual disturbances. On examination you note a blue-grey discoloration of his skin.
3. An 83-year-old man with a history of hypertension presents with a dry cough. Routine blood investigations demonstrate a potassium of 6 mmol/L.
4. A 59-year-old woman with a history of hypertension presents to the GP for a routine blood test. Results demonstrate a sodium of 129 mmol/L and a potassium of 6.3 mmol/L.
5. A 45-year-old man recently commenced on an antihypertensive presents with a hot swollen right toe.

Question 2
a) Lisinopril
b) Candesartan
c) Amlodipine
d) Amiodarone
e) Glyceryl trinitrate (GTN)
f) Atenolol
g) Bisoprolol
h) Isosorbide mononitrate
i) Nicorandil

For each patient below, what is the most appropriate treatment option?
Select ONE option only from the list above.
Each option may be selected once, more than once or not at all.

1. A 43-year-old man with congestive cardiac failure presents with shortness of breath. A chest X-ray on arrival demonstrates evidence of an enlarged heart and pulmonary congestion. He is given 80 mg furosemide intravenously. An hour later his breathing becomes more

laboured. Routine observations reveal a pulse rate of 105 beats per minute and a blood pressure of 110/75 mmHg.

2. A 62-year-old Caucasian man is reviewed by his GP. His blood pressure is 192/75 mmHg on three separate readings. Current medication includes aspirin 75 mg and bendroflumethiazide 2.5 mg.

3. A 53-year-old Caucasian woman presents to her GP for a routine check-up. Her blood pressure is noted to be 165/94 mmHg on three separate readings. Current medication includes aspirin 75 mg.

4. A 45-year-old woman presents with a dry cough. She has a background history of hypertension and is currently on ramipril 5 mg.

5. A 78-year-old man presents to his GP for a routine check-up. He has a background history of hypertension. Current medication includes bendroflumethiazide and ramipril. His blood pressure is still elevated at 175/105 mmHg.

Question 3

a) Lisinopril
b) Indapamide
c) Minoxidil
d) Clonidine
e) Losartan
f) Felodipine
g) Propranolol
h) Hydralazine
i) Doxazosin

For each patient below, what is the most likely cause?
Select ONE option only from the list above.
Each option may be selected once, more than once or not at all.

1. A 72-year-old woman is admitted to the Emergency Department with gradual-onset swelling of her eyes and lips. She is a known hypertensive patient and has been started on a new medication recently.

2. A 63-year-old man presents with soreness of his gums. He has a history of high blood pressure. On examination you note evidence of gingival hyperplasia.

3. A 69-year-old man presents with generalised joint pains. On examination you note evidence of an erythematous rash on his face which he comments gets worse in sunlight.

4. A 62-year-old woman registers at her local GP practice. She is a known hypertensive and undergoes a medication review. During the consultation you note evidence of fine, dark-coloured hair on her face and arms.

5. A 56-year-old man with a background history of chronic obstructive pulmonary disease (COPD) has been recently started on a new tablet for his blood pressure. He is admitted to the Emergency Department with increasing shortness of breath. He denies any cough or fever.

Answers

Single best answer questions

Q1 d.

Mitral stenosis has several causes including rheumatic fever, systemic lupus erythematosus and rheumatoid arthritis. Symptoms include exertional dyspnoea, orthopnoea and, in severe cases, pulmonary oedema. The murmur is classically heard as a low-pitched rumbling diastolic murmur over the apex. Mitral regurgitation results in a high-pitched blowing murmur over the apex which may radiate to the left axilla. Aortic stenosis results in an ejection systolic murmur in the second right intercostal space that radiates to the carotids. Pulmonary stenosis is associated with a systolic ejection murmur in the left upper sternal border that increases with inspiration. Aortic regurgitation is a diastolic murmur that is high-pitched and loudest at the left sternal border.

Q2 d.

In accordance with NICE guidelines, hypertensive patients aged 55 or over or Afro-Caribbean patients should be commenced on a calcium channel blocker or thiazide diuretic. Those younger than 55 should be commenced on an angiotensin converting enzyme (ACE) inhibitor or an angiotensin II receptor antagonist if an ACE inhibitor is not tolerated.

Q3 b.

From the history and cardiac risk factors the most likely diagnosis is an acute coronary syndrome. Hence an ECG as a first-line investigation is paramount. The other investigations are all of relevance but would not be deemed as the most important in this scenario. Patients presenting with cardiac-sounding chest pain should be 'TIMI' (thrombolysis in myocardial infarction) scored to assess their mortality risk. The score comprises the following criteria:

Age > 65 years
> 3 risk factors for coronary artery disease
Known coronary artery disease > 50% stenosis
ASA use in past 7 days
Severe angina
ST changes > 0.5 mm
Positive cardiac marker

Q4 c.

Pericarditis is associated with inflammation of the pericardium. It presents with chest pain which may be sharp or dull and exacerbated during inspiration and when lying flat. Concave ST elevation is diagnostic of the condition. Examination findings may include a pericardial rub which is scratching in character. Causes of pericarditis are numerous and include tuberculosis, systemic lupus erythematosus, rheumatoid arthritis, renal failure, hypothyroidism, streptococcus and coxsackievirus B. The management of pericarditis includes NSAIDs in the main.

Q5 a.
Hypertrophic cardiomyopathy is a genetic autosomal dominant condition associated typically with hypertrophy of the left ventricle and resulting in blood flow obstruction. It can result in sudden cardiac death, dyspnoea, syncope and presyncope. Pulmonary embolism results typically in pleuritic chest pain, shortness of breath and haemoptysis. Significant risk factors include a previous history of venous thromboembolism, recent surgery, oestrogen use, cancer and reduced mobility. Aortic dissection is associated with tearing type chest pain which can radiate to the back. Blood pressure may vary inter-arm in up to 30% of cases. Commotio cordis is sudden cardiac death that occurs following a non-penetrating blow to the chest. Studies have shown that an impact typically over the left ventricle may result in ventricular fibrillation and subsequent death.

Q6 e.
These are the classic ECG findings of Wolff-Parkinson-White syndrome. Treatment of choice includes adenosine or procainamide. Vasovagal syncope presents with dizzy spells, palpitations, nausea and sweating. It is typically cardiac, orthostatic or neurological in nature. First-degree heart block is associated with a prolonged PR interval on the ECG. Atrial fibrillation is associated with an irregular ventricular rate and absent P waves.

Q7 b.
Contraindications from the American College of Cardiology/American Heart Association include:

Myocardial infarction
Unstable angina
Aortic stenosis
Heart failure
Pulmonary embolism
Myocarditis
Aortic dissection
Left main coronary artery stenosis
Electrolyte abnormalities
Hypertrophic cardiomyopathy
Mental or physical impairment

Q8 a.
The ECG is most likely a supraventricular tachycardia (SVT) which is best treated with adenosine. An irregular narrow complex tachycardia is most likely atrial fibrillation which would require a beta-blocker or diltiazem for rate control.

Q9 d.

In accordance with advanced life support (ALS) guidelines a tachycardia with adverse features such as shock, syncope, myocardial ischaemia and heart failure is best treated by a synchronised DC shock. At least three attempts are made, followed by amiodarone intravenously.

Q10 a.

Dressler's syndrome is a form of pericarditis that is seen following a myocardial infarction. Treatment of choice includes NSAIDs. Pneumonia typically presents with shortness of breath, productive cough and a fever. Cardiac tamponade is associated with chest pain and fatigue. Examination findings include an increased jugular venous pressure, hypotension and diminished heart sounds (Beck's triad).

Q11 e.

Acute coronary syndrome is treated with aspirin 300 mg, clopidogrel 300 mg, enoxaparin 1 mg/kg and bisoprolol 5 mg. A statin, typically atorvastatin, is also of importance.

Q12 e.

An urgent coronary angiography would be most suitable as it would help to localise cardiac vessel stenosis which would be amenable to stenting. An acute coronary syndrome is a contraindication to exercise treadmill testing. A dobutamine stress echo is utilised when individuals are unable to exercise on a treadmill and require assessment of cardiac function.

Q13 a.

Spironolactone is a potassium-sparing diuretic. Side effects include a high potassium and low sodium. Additional side effects include gastrointestinal bleeding, gynaecomastia and ataxia. Bumetanide and furosemide are loop diuretics and result in a low serum sodium and potassium. Bendroflumethiazide results in hyperuricaemia, hypokalaemia, hypophosphataemia and hypomagnesaemia.

Q14 e.

Risperidone is an antipsychotic that can precipitate long QT syndrome. It presents as syncope and in severe cases cardiac arrest. Sick sinus syndrome is associated with dizziness, syncope and palpitations. An ECG is likely to demonstrate sinus bradycardia with sinus pauses.

Q15 a.

Type I hyperlipoproteinaemia presents with abdominal pain secondary to pancreatitis. The white discoloration of the retina is termed lipemia retinalis. Xanthomas and hepatosplenomegaly are common. The treatment of choice is dietary control. The condition is associated with increased chylomicrons and decreased lipoprotein lipase.

Extended matching questions
Question 1
Q1 e.
Amlodipine is a calcium channel antagonist, commonly associated with ankle swelling. Additional side effects include sweating, a dry mouth, headaches, hot flushes and palpitations.

Q2 h.
Amiodarone commonly causes pulmonary fibrosis. In addition it can lead to corneal microdeposits and a disorder of thyroid function. Patients may complain of seeing a bluish halo, and a blue-grey skin discoloration.

Q3 c.
Ramipril is an ACE inhibitor that can result in renal impairment. A dry cough is common as well as hypoglycaemia, nausea and a yellow discoloration of the skin or eyes.

Q4 d.
Spironolactone is an aldosterone antagonist which results in a low sodium and high potassium. Additional side effects include muscle weakness, bradycardia and breast enlargement commonly in men.

Q5 f.
Bendroflumethiazide is a thiazide diuretic. It can result in hyperuricaemia and subsequently gout. Additional side effects include dizziness and abdominal discomfort.

Question 2
Q1 e.
Worsening heart failure that is not responding to furosemide should be treated with a trial of glyceryl trinitrate (GTN) infusion to help offload the heart as long as the blood pressure remains stable.

Q2 a.
In accordance with NICE guidelines, patients aged 55 or more or black patients of any age should be commenced on a calcium channel blocker or thiazide diuretic. If there is no improvement in blood pressure while on the latter, an ACE inhibitor should be added.

Q3 a.
In accordance with NICE guidelines, patients younger than 55 years of age should be commenced on an ACE inhibitor if hypertensive.

Q4 b.
ACE inhibitors are associated with a dry cough due to inhibition of bradykinin metabolism. An alternative therapy therefore is an angiotensin II receptor antagonist such as candesartan which does not result in a cough.

Q5 c.

In accordance with NICE guidelines, patients with hypertension over the age of 55 or who are of black descent should be commenced on a calcium channel blocker or thiazide diuretic initially. If the patient fails to respond, an ACE inhibitor is added. If there is no response to both an ACE inhibitor and thiazide diuretic then a calcium channel blocker is added.

Question 3

Q1 a.

ACE inhibitors are known to cause a dry cough, renal impairment and angioedema.

Q2 f.

Calcium channel blockers are commonly associated with gum hyperplasia and hypertrophy.

Q3 h.

Hydralazine can induce lupus erythematosus. Additional side effects include diarrhoea, a compensatory tachycardia, headaches and depression.

Q4 c.

Minoxidil is commonly associated with excessive hair growth. It is a potassium channel activator and has been used for the treatment of hypertension. Additional side effects include visual disturbance, chest pain and pseudoacromegaly.

Q5 g.

Beta-blockers are associated with bronchospasm and hence should be avoided in those with COPD and asthma.

2 Dermatology

For each question below, what is the most likely answer?
Select ONE option only from the answers supplied.

1. You are an F2 doctor and have been called to the Emergency
    Department to see a 4-year-old girl with a diffuse rash all over her
    body; the rash is erythematous and non-blanching with discrete lesions.
    She has a high fever and appears drowsy. What is the most likely
    diagnosis?
    a) Meningococcal infection
    b) Henoch–Schönlein purpura
    c) Varicella zoster
    d) Herpes simplex
    e) Rubella

2. You are working in a rheumatology post and you are asked to see a
    42-year-old woman with rheumatoid arthritis. Which one of these
    conditions is commonly associated with rheumatoid arthritis?
    a) Violacious rash
    b) Sclerodactyly
    c) Butterfly rash
    d) Raynaud syndrome
    e) Erythema nodosum

3. A 37-year-old woman is diagnosed with sarcoidosis. What skin
    manifestation might you expect to see?
    a) Erythema marginatum
    b) Erythema chronicum migrans
    c) Erythema multiforme
    d) Erythema nodosum

The Complete GPVTS Stage 2 Preparation Guide: Questions and Professional Dilemmas,
First Edition. Edited by Saba Khan with Neel Sharma.
© 2012 John Wiley & Sons, Ltd. Published 2012 by John Wiley & Sons, Ltd.

4. A 72-year-old man presents with shingles (Herpes zoster) in the Emergency Department. When are antivirals recommended?
   a) Within 2 weeks
   b) Within 72 hours
   c) Within 10 days
   d) Within 48 hours
   e) Within 24 hours

5. You are an F2 doctor in general practice, and are asked to see a 15-year-old boy with mild acne. What is the first-line treatment option?
   a) Oral isotretinoin
   b) Topical isotretinoin
   c) Oral cyproterone acetate
   d) Oral tetracycline
   e) Topical benzoyl peroxide + clindamycin

6. You are asked to see an 18-year-old girl with genital warts in the genitourinary medicine (GUM) clinic. What are the two most common treatment options?
   a) Imiquimod cream
   b) Cryotherapy with/without podophyllin
   c) Intralesional interferon
   d) Topical steroids
   e) Griseofulvin

7. A 22-year-old man presents with a round, scaly, itchy lesion with an inflamed edge and central sparing on his torso. What is the most likely diagnosis?
   a) Pityriasis rosea
   b) Pityriasis alba
   c) Pityriasis versicolor
   d) Tinea
   e) Psoriasis

8. An 18-year-old girl presents with a widespread erythematous discrete blanching rash over her torso and back, with a 'christmas-tree distribution'. What is the most likely diagnosis?
   a) Pityriasis alba
   b) Pityriasis rosea
   c) Pityriasis versicolor
   d) Pityriasis rubra pilaris
   e) Pityriasis lichenoides

9. Which one of the following conditions does NOT cause generalised itching?
   a) Hyper/hypothyroidism
   b) Chronic renal failure
   c) Chronic liver disease

d) Chronic heart failure

e) Lymphoma

10. Which of these is NOT premalignant?
   a) Lentigo maligna
   b) Halo naevus
   c) Actinic keratosis
   d) Bowen disease

11. Which one of these conditions is NOT associated with systemic lupus erythematosus?
   a) Butterfly rash
   b) Discoid rash
   c) Photosensitivity
   d) Oral ulcers
   e) Lupus pernio

12. Which of these is NOT associated with sarcoidosis?
   a) Erythema nodosum
   b) Lupus pernio
   c) Subcutaneous nodules
   d) Conjunctivitis
   e) Erythema migrans

13. Which two of the following causes scarring alopecia?
   a) Iron/zinc deficiency
   b) Childbirth
   c) Lichen planus
   d) Alopecia areata
   e) Discoid lupus erythematosus

14. Which one of the following is NOT a common cause of urticaria?
   a) Shellfish
   b) Strawberries
   c) Rice
   d) Eggs
   e) Chocolates

15. Which one of the following is NOT a common skin manifestation of HIV?
   a) Molluscum contagiosum
   b) Varicella zoster
   c) Scabies
   d) Pityriasis rosea
   e) Oral hairy leukoplakia

Extended matching questions

Question 1
a) Necrobiosis lipoidica
b) Erythema nodosum
c) Target lesions
d) Dermatitis herpetiformis
e) Butterfly rash
f) Lupus pernio
g) Sclerodactyly
h) Alopecia
i) Heliotrope rash
j) Acanthosis nigricans
k) Pyoderma gangrenosum
l) Angular chelitis
m) Folliculitis
n) Neurofibroma

1. Which one of the above conditions is most likely to present in a 21-year-old female with insulin-dependent diabetes?
2. Which two skin manifestations are found in patients with systemic lupus erythematosus?
3. A 64-year-old man is diagnosed with advanced stomach cancer. Which one of these skin manifestations could his condition most likely to be associated with?

Question 2
a) Basal cell carcinoma (BCC)
b) Squamous cell carcinoma (SCC)
c) Bowen disease
d) Actinic keratoses
e) Malignant melanoma
f) Mycosis fungoides
g) Paget disease
h) Pyoderma gangrenosum
i) Lichen planus
j) Hypertrichosis lanuginosa
k) Telangiectasia
l) Lentigo maligna
m) Granuloma annulare

1. Which one of the above conditions follows a benign, self-limiting course?
2. Which one of these conditions requires urgent referral to a breast surgeon?
3. Which two of the above conditions would need urgent referral to a dermatologist?

Question 3

a) Tar
b) Vitamin D analogues (calcipotriol)
c) Hydrocortisone 1%
d) Betamethasone
e) Fusidic acid
f) Methotrexate
g) Phototherapy
h) Infliximab
i) Emollients
j) Tacrolimus
k) Terbinafine
l) Selenium sulfide shampoo
m) Imidazole cream
n) Education
o) Metronidazole gel

1. What topical treatment from the above list can be used as a steroid sparing agent in patients with eczema over the age of two?
2. Which two topical treatments are used in psoriasis, for long-term control of the condition and improving quality of life?
3. Which one of the above treatments is most suitable for fungal nail infections?

Answers

Single best answer questions

Q1 a.

Meningitis needs to be diagnosed quickly and treated as soon as possible. Local protocols can vary, but intravenous antibiotics are given in hospital followed by dexamethasone. In the community setting if signs of meningism are present then intramuscular benzylpenicillin should be administered.

Q2 d.

Raynaud syndrome occurs as a result of exposure to cold with colour changes to the skin: first white (ischaemia), then blue (deoxygenation) and then red (reperfusion). Digits are painful and symptoms can be brought on by stress and cold. Raynaud disease (idiopathic) or Raynaud phenomenon (underlying cause) is helped by keeping the hands warm and stopping smoking. Nifedipine, losartan, prazosin and fluoxetine have been shown to help. Sympathectomy in more severe cases can be tried.

Q3 d.

Sarcoid is a multisystem granulomatous disorder. It is more common in young adults and can present with vague chest discomfort. The disease can run an acute course with hilar lymph node involvement or a more chronic course with multisystem involvement. Up to 90% of patients can spontaneously recover, but those with more persistent disease can be treated with corticosteroids.

Q4 b.

It is recommended to start treatment at the latest within 72 hours in order for there to be treatment benefit. If treated in time, patients have been shown to have reduced length of rash and less acute pain.

Q5 e.

First-line treatment in patients with mild acne consists of topical keratolytics and antiseptics. Topical antibiotics can also be used alone or in combination therapies.

Q6 a, b.

Patients can be treated in clinic or can be given treatment to take home with them.

Imiquimod is an immune response modifier, and in some women has been shown to completely clear the warts. The patient's partner should also be seen and treated as necessary. In addition, patients should be screened for other STIs.

Patients are advised to use barrier contraception in order to avoid pregnancy and to prevent further transmission.

Q7 d.
Tinea corporis is a common fungal skin infection. Single annular lesions develop with central sparing and an erythematous raised edge. Lesions are best treated with topical imidazole creams; in more severe cases oral antifungals can be used.

Q8 b.
Piyriasis rosea is an acute, self-limiting condition following a viral infection. More prolonged episodes can occur following some drug therapies.

Q9 d.
High levels of urea and bilirubin can cause generalised pruritus as can thyroid dysfunction, and pruritus can be the presenting feature of Hodgkin lymphoma. Patients should have a careful history taken and blood testing, including FBC, U&E function and LFTs.

Q10 b.
Halo naevi generally occur at the time of puberty. They are naevi that involute from an immunological rejection mechanism, and as such during the involution process are surrounded by a ring of paler skin. This is not a premalignant condition but has an association with melanoma and such patients should be thoroughly examined for lesions.

Q11 e.
Lupus pernio is a cutaneous manifestation of sarcoid disease. It takes the form of blue-red nodules that can develop on the face, hands or nose.

Q12 e.
Erythema migrans is the skin lesion that develops approximately 1 week to 10 days after a bite from the *Ixodes* genus tick which is the cause of Lyme disease. The lesion spreads to form an annular lesion with central sparing.

Q13 c, e.
In non-scarring alopecia hair follicles are not damaged and hair loss can resolve completely. Scarring alopecia causes destruction of the hair follicles and therefore permanent hair loss. Other causes of scarring alopecia are trauma, lichen sclerosus and localised scleroderma.

Q14 c.
Urticaria is a vascular reaction of the skin, which is characterised by raised pale swellings on the skin associated with intense itching.

Urticaria is caused by certain foods, infections, drugs and also emotional stress. Physical triggers include heat, cold, exercise or touch.

Q15 d.
Pityriasis rosea is a rash with a characteristic Christmas-tree distribution across the torso. It is brought on by a viral infection and is generally self-limiting.

The remaining conditions are all associations of HIV, as HIV-positive patients are more prone to infections caused by organisms which do not usually cause infection in immuno-competent adults. These common conditions are often more florid and severe in their presentation.

Extended matching questions
Question 1
Q1 a.

Necrobiosis lipoidica is a lesion commonly found on the anterior aspect of the shin, as a waxy brown plaque. It is three times as common in women than in men, and tends to present in young adults.

Q2 e, h.

Systemic lupus erythematosus is a multisystemic autoimmune condition. The main clinical symptoms are fever, malaise, weight loss and tiredness. There is no single diagnostic test for systemic lupus erythematosus, rather diagnosis is made by the presence of at least four criteria out of eleven, proposed by the American Rheumatism Association.

Q3 j.

Acanthosis nigricans is characterised by brown/black hyperpigmentation of the skin, specifically in the axillary, inframammary and inguinal areas. It is also associated with endocrine disorders and obesity.

Question 2
Q1 m.

Granuloma annulare is characterised by dermal nodules that develop in a circular formation. It can be seen in all ages, and gradually enlarges over time. It is associated with diabetes mellitus in adults.

The condition is self-limiting but can take some months to resolve.

Q2 g.

Paget disease of the nipple appears as a unilateral eczematous discrete area of skin, that can bleed, and does not resolve with standard treatments. It is typically associated with underlying ductal carcinoma of the breast.

Q3 b, e.

Both malignant melanoma and squamous cell carcinoma require urgent referral due to the high metastatic and erosive potential of both conditions.

Question 3
Q1 j.

Tacrolimus can be used topically in children over the age of two, when steroids have failed or skin thinning has occurred. It can be applied sparingly twice daily under dermatological supervision.

Q2 b, d.

Vitamin D analogues and steroids are used in combination for reducing the psoriasis and good symptom control. Other agents such as coal tar are also effective but are more difficult to use.

Q3 k.

Terbinafine is the recommended treatment in fungal nail infections for a period of 3 months. During the course of treatment, blood testing for liver function should be carried out to monitor the possibility of side effects.

3 Ear, Nose and Throat

For each question below, what is the most likely answer?
Select one or more options only from the answers supplied.

1. A patient presents with Bell's palsy, following an acute viral infection. Which are the two treatment options?
   a) Steroids
   b) High-dose acyclovir
   c) Tricyclic antidepressants
   d) Carbamazepine
   e) Acupuncture

2. Which of the following factors are NOT true of oesophageal cancer?
   a) Smokers are at an increased risk
   b) Early treatment with proton pump inhibitors (PPIs) can prevent disease progression
   c) Post resection, patients have a good 5-year survival rate
   d) Patients with Barrett's oesophagus require regular endoscopic surveillance
   e) There is an association with iron deficiency anaemia

3. Hoarseness is often the only presenting feature of laryngeal cancer, and should be investigated if it persists after which time frame?
   a) 1 week
   b) 2 weeks
   c) 3 weeks
   d) 6 weeks
   e) 6 months

4. Singers' nodules are best treated with which treatment option?
   a) Surgery
   b) Speech therapy

The Complete GPVTS Stage 2 Preparation Guide: Questions and Professional Dilemmas,
First Edition. Edited by Saba Khan with Neel Sharma.
© 2012 John Wiley & Sons, Ltd. Published 2012 by John Wiley & Sons, Ltd.

   c) Conservative management
   d) Broad-spectrum antibiotics
   e) Complete voice rest

5. Which of the following statements are true of hypothyroidism?
   a) Free T3 is reduced and T4 is raised
   b) Is caused by a thyroid adenoma
   c) Is usually treated with liothyronine
   d) Can result following treatment for hyperthyroidism
   e) Treatment requires blood testing every 3 months

6. Otitis media is best treated by which one of the following treatments?
   a) Oral antibiotics
   b) Topical antibiotics
   c) Analgesia
   d) Decongestants
   e) Grommets

7. Features of temporomandibular joint dysfunction include which two of the following?
   a) Sore throat
   b) Facial pain
   c) Tinnitus
   d) Earache
   e) Vomiting

8. Glue ear is more frequently found in which one of the following?
   a) Girls
   b) Cold weather
   c) Down syndrome
   d) Post tonsillectomy
   e) Children over the age of 5

9. Which one of the following factors can cause a conductive hearing loss?
   a) Congenital cholesteatoma
   b) Toxoplasmosis
   c) Ototoxic drugs
   d) Turner syndrome
   e) Hyperbilirubinaemia

10. Sudden hearing loss is associated with which two of the following?
   a) Measles
   b) Mumps
   c) Noise exposure
   d) Age over 50
   e) Rubella

11. Xerostomia is NOT a feature in which two conditions?
    a) Hypothyroidism
    b) Sjögren syndrome
    c) Antipsychotic medication
    d) Sinusitis
    e) Tricyclic antidepressants

12. Bell's palsy is associated with which cranial nerve?
    a) CN II
    b) CN III
    c) CN V
    d) CN VI
    e) CNVII

13. Which one of the following does NOT cause hearing loss?
    a) Rheumatoid arthritis
    b) Gout
    c) Ankylosing spondylitis
    d) Systemic sclerosis
    e) Systemic lupus erythematosus

14. Which is the most common form of thyroid cancer?
    a) Anaplastic
    b) Medullary
    c) Papillary
    d) Lymphoma
    e) Follicular

15. In which of the following clinical scenarios would you NOT
    recommend surgery for thyroid removal?
    a) Relapsing hyperthyroidism following failed drug treatment
    b) Symptomatic hyperthyroid patients prior to planning pregnancy
    c) Cosmetic reasons
    d) Family history of thyroid cancer
    e) Pressure symptoms from thyroid enlargement

Extended matching questions

Question 1
Which of the following are most suitable responses in the following scenarios?
a) Boys
b) Turner syndrome
c) Down syndrome
d) Audiogram
e) Girls
f) Community audiology service
g) Conductive hearing loss
h) Sensorineural hearing loss
i) Otoacoustic emissions testing
j) Distraction testing
k) Conditioned response audiometry
l) Pure tone audiogram
m) ENT referral

1. A 2-year-old child presents with hearing loss for a period of 4 weeks, reported by his mother. Where should the child be referred and what would be the most appropriate investigation for him?
2. A mother brings her 3-year-old son to her GP as she has been worried for the last 6 months that her son is not responding to her when she calls him. She explains that he has had repeated ear infections and has been deteriorating in his behaviour. What is the most appropriate referral for him and what is his most likely diagnosis?
3. A baby is born with lymphoedema of the feet, a webbed neck and low-set ears. What is the most likely diagnosis and which type of hearing loss is most common?

Question 2
Choose the most appropriate responses to the following questions.
a) Oesophageal carcinoma
b) Achalasia
c) Pharyngeal carcinoma
d) Nasopharyngeal cancer
e) Laryngomalacia
f) Benign oesophageal stricture
g) Barrett's oesophagus
h) Acoustic neuroma
i) Croup
j) Laryngeal paralysis
k) Retropharyngeal abscess
l) Peritonsillar abcess (quinsy)
m) Laryngeal nerve palsy

1. A 68-year-old man presents with a persistent left-sided ear effusion, and reduced hearing on the same side. He also has had epistaxis on the same side over the last few months which he has never experienced before. The symptoms have been present for many months now; it is difficult to elicit the history as English is not his first language. The history is taken via an interpreter who speaks fluent Chinese. What is his most likely diagnosis?

2. A 24-year-old man presents with a 2-week history of sore throat, fever and sweating. He has presented to the Emergency Department out of hours because he has severe pain on the right side of his throat which has slowly worsened over the last day; he feels he cannot even swallow his own saliva. What is the most likely diagnosis?

3. A 35-year-old woman presents with difficulty swallowing both liquids and solids; she finds it takes her a long time to swallow anything. She has had no weight loss and has a normal appetite. She explains that her symptoms have been developing over a very long time, perhaps years. What is the most likely diagnosis?

Question 3

Choose the most appropriate response from the following list:

a) Amoxicillin
b) Analgesia
c) Betahistine
d) Computed tomography scan
e) Intravenous antibiotics
f) Grommets
g) Xylometazoline
h) Cyclizine
i) Beclometasone
j) Prednisolone
k) Cochlear implants
l) No treatment
m) Nortriptyline
n) Cetirizine
o) Fluticasone
p) Topical lidocaine

1. An 18-year-old with recurrent epistaxis presents at the Emergency Department with a nose bleed that has already lasted half an hour; the bleeding is quite profuse and the patient explains this is worse than usual. The patient has been playing football outside and was hit in the face, and has been using Nurofen for an ankle injury. Which two treatments would you use in this patient?

2. A 42-year-old woman presents with symptoms of the room spinning, tinnitus and hearing loss in the right ear. She explains that the dizziness has made her feel nauseous and has led to two episodes of vomiting. What are the two treatments that could be tried in this patient?

3. A 10-month-old child is brought in by her mother with an acute ear infection. The child has a history of recurrent ear infections; however, on this occasion, the child has a fever and the mother reports that she seems more unwell than usual. Examination reveals acute otitis media, with generalised malaise and fever. No other worrying features are present. What is the best management for this patient?

Answers

Single best answer questions

Q1 a, b.

Bell's palsy is a lower motor neurone palsy with abrupt onset resulting in complete unilateral facial weakness. Presentation is with facial distortion, dribbling, taste impairment, hyperacusis and a watery or dry eye from failure of eyelid closure. It is more common in pregnancy and diabetes.

Treatment is with protection of the eye, followed by steroids preferably within 24 hours as this offers the most benefit. High-dose antiviral agents are given where a viral cause such as herpes zoster is suspected.

Q2 c.

Oesophageal cancer is more common in men by a five to one ratio; it is associated with alcohol excess, smoking, reflux oesophagitis and Barrett's oesophagus, as well as obesity and diet. The survival rates are low with or without treatment and post resection survival rates are also poor. A palliative approach is preferred in advanced disease.

Q3 c.

Hoarseness is the main and often only presentation of laryngeal carcinoma; if persistent for more than 3 weeks, investigation is needed to rule out more serious disease. There are many benign causes of a hoarse voice, the most common of which are gastro-oesophageal reflux and voice over-use.

Q4 b.

Singers' nodules typically occur in patients who use their voice more than others, such as singers and teachers. They are small benign swellings on the opposing surfaces of the true cords. The swellings occur as the vocal cords are constantly banging together. Small nodules can be treated with speech therapy, though larger nodules are reviewed for surgical removal.

Q5 d.

Hypothyroidism is characterised by lethargy, weight gain and slowness as the presenting features in adults, and as a result of this, presentation maybe after some years. Patients are usually in their 50s or 60s. Causes are primary or secondary, with primary causes arising from the gland itself and secondary from deficiency of the stimulating factors for the thyroid. Treatment is with lifelong thyroxine therapy at doses titrated until patients are euthyroid. Once this dose is reached, patients are left on a maintenance dose.

Q6 c.

The vast majority of middle ear infections clear within 3 days without any management. Over-the-counter (OTC) analgesia is often the only treatment needed to relieve discomfort and reduce fever in patients.

Antibiotics are considered in patients under the age of 2, those who are systemically unwell or children with recurrent infections.

Q7 b, d.
Temporomandibular joint dysfunction can be as a result of the musculature, displacement of the joint itself or from arthritis. The pain from temporomandibular mandibular joint dysfunction will often resolve simultaneously with a soft diet and analgesia; specific causes are treated. Other features include jaw pain, headache, neck stiffness and tinnitus.

Q8 b, c.
Glue ear or secretory otitis media is caused by accumulation of fluid in the middle ear, resulting in pain and conductive hearing loss.

Most cases resolve within 3 months though a small minority can persist to a year with hearing loss. It is more common in children aged 2–5, in boys, children with Down syndrome and in those children exposed to cigarette smoke. Treatment is with referral for audiometry/medication and assessment for grommet surgery.

Q9 a.
Conductive hearing loss results from any disruption of sound waves reaching the ear drum or free movement of the drum and its apparatus. This contrasts to sensorineural hearing loss which is as a result of damage to the vestibulocochlear nerve.

Q10 b, c.
Sudden hearing loss requires immediate referral to a specialist for assessment and management. Noise exposure leads to damage of the hair cells in the cochlea and mumps is also a cause of damage to the cochlea though only a small proportion of mumps patients develop permanent hearing loss.

Q11 a, d.
Xerostomia or dry mouth can result from drugs (hypnotics, tricyclics, antipsychotics, beta-blockers and diuretics), mouth breathing, dehydration, radiotherapy, systemic lupus erythematosus, scleroderma, HIV and sarcoid.

Q12 e.
Bell's palsy is usually caused by entrapment of the seventh cranial nerve leading to inflammatory oedema of the nerve, commonly resulting from latent herpes infection. This results in the clinical picture of a lower motor neurone lesion in the face. CN 2, 3 and 6 are normally associated with eye movements. Cranial nerve 5 is associated with the motor function of the facial muscles.

Q13 b.
Gout can cause tophi on the helix of the outer ear. The remaining autoimmune conditions are all associated with varying presentations of sensorineural hearing loss.

Q14 c.

Papillary carcinoma is the most common thyroid cancer, making up the majority of cases, followed by follicular cancer. Medullary and lymphoma types are rare and anaplastic cancer is the least common. Papillary and follicular cancers are differentiated cancers usually treated with surgery and radiotherapy. Medullary cancers tend to occur in familial cases, with lymphoma and anaplastic cancer being more common in the elderly.

Q15 d.

In familial thyroid cancers, both sexes are equally affected, and the age of onset is variable. Familial cases have an autosomal dominant inheritance, they are bilateral and multifocal. Surgical thyroid removal is not recommended prophylactically unless part of the MEN II syndrome.

Extended matching questions
Question 1
Q1 f, k.

The community audiology referral will help to find out what kind of hearing loss is present and also if there is any resulting impairment; given the short history this is not an unreasonable plan. If the hearing loss had been for a longer period of time then a direct ENT referral would have been more suitable. The patient's age predetermines which sort of testing is most appropriate; in this case, conditioned response audiometry is best. This method requires the child to follow a simple instruction in response to specific auditory cues; it is the most age-appropriate option.

Q2 m, g.

In this case the patient has a much longer history, as well as resulting behavioural change and potential delay in development. In this instance it would be more appropriate to refer to ENT for an opinion as to the best course of management. The patient is likely to have glue ear and hence would have a conductive hearing loss as a consequence of build-up of fluid behind the ear drum.

Q3 b, h.

The clinical features described are those of Turner syndrome. The condition is caused by the 45 XO karyotype, and occurs in approx 1 in 2500 births. It is also characterised by a broad shield chest and wide-spaced nipples, low hairline, short fourth metacarpal and cubitus valgus. These patients can also have sensorineural hearing loss.

Question 2
Q1 d.

Nasopharyngeal cancer is a poorly differentiated cancer that appears on the lateral wall of the nasopharynx near the ostium of the eustachian tube. It is more common in people of Chinese-Asian descent.

Patients typically present with deafness, epistaxis or bilateral cervical node involvement. Symptoms will then develop dependent on spread and invasion of disease. These can involve the cranial nerves, affecting functions of the nose, ear, eye or pharynx.

Patients are investigated with biopsy and imaging, followed by intensive radiotherapy which has been shown to improve 5-year survival rates.

Q2 l.
Quinsy is a complication of acute tonsillitis. Tonsillitis is commonly caused by streptococcal infection. The quinsy is a collection of pus adherent to the tonsil.

Patients are treated with penicillin, or erythromycin if allergic to penicillin. The quinsy is incised and drained to remove the pus; patients are then followed up for possible tonsillectomy.

Q3 b.
This is a condition that develops from failure of the lower part of the oesophagus to dilate, hindering passage of food and fluid. Over time this causes dilatation of the oesophagus above the area of constriction and also dysfunctional motility along the oesophagus, impairing peristalsis.

Achalasia is associated with a greater risk of oesophageal malignancy but this is likely to be as a result of prolonged food transit and hence prolonged exposure of the oesophagus to different agents.

Patients can be treated by botulinum toxin to relax the lower third of the muscle wall, or the muscle wall can be dilated using balloon dilatation. This procedure would need frequent repetition, whereas the surgical option is a cardiomyotomy to open up the muscle wall permanently. Each method has its own complication rate and patients need to be counselled about these.

Question 3
Q1 g, p.
Epistaxis is a common condition that generally occurs in the very young or very old. If it occurs outside these age ranges then it is more likely to be as a result of trauma or more serious disease. The point of bleeding is usually Little's area, which is the anterior blood supply. Patients can usually be managed conservatively by tipping the head forward and pressing over the bridge of the nose to apply pressure to the septal area. Patients can also use ice packs which can help to reduce blood flow.

Xylometazoline is a vasoconstrictor and lidocaine is a local anaesthetic; these two agents can be applied to the septal area using gauze. This is done in patients in whom bleeding is not controlled by conservative measures.

Q2 c, h.
Meniere disease is the condition described in this scenario and is made up of this classic triad of symptoms. Usually only one ear is affected, in

which patients can describe a feeling of fullness. They also can have nausea and vomiting. The aetiology of this condition is not known, hence investigations are based on hearing levels and balance testing.

During an acute attack patients are advised to sit still and to use antiemetics until symptoms pass; betahistine can be used to alleviate symptoms though the evidence for its use is limited.

Patients that have clusters of attacks that do not respond to medical management can be referred for surgical decompression of the endolymphatic sac. More invasive techniques are also available but patients should be fully counselled and disease severity assessed.

Q3 a.
The general advice for patients with acute otitis media is that the condition is often viral and therefore self-limiting. However, in some patients where the age of the child is under 2 years, systemic features are present or if the patient suffers from recurrent infections, antibiotics can be trialled to prevent further complications. The evidence for withholding or treating with antibiotics does still however point toward withholding antibiotics in most patients presenting with acute otitis media.

4 Endocrinology and Metabolic Disease

For each question below, what is the most likely answer?
Select ONE option only from the answers supplied.

1. A 48-year-old woman presents to her GP. She comments that she has been feeling particularly dizzy over the past one month. She denies any weakness or numbness of any kind. On examination you note a blood pressure of 85/48 mmHg. You observe evidence of pigmentation of her skin creases. What is the most likely diagnosis?
   a) Nelson's syndrome
   b) Addison's disease
   c) Sheehan's syndrome
   d) Kallman's syndrome
   e) Cushing's syndrome

2. A 23-year-old man is admitted to hospital. On examination you note he is obese with stretch marks on his abdomen in addition to thinning of his skin. He comments that he has particular difficult climbing stairs. What is the most likely diagnosis?
   a) Polymyositis
   b) Addison's disease
   c) Sheehan's syndrome
   d) Cushing's syndrome
   e) Nelson's syndrome

3. A 34-year-old woman presents to her GP. She complains of difficulties in menstruating following a traumatic childbirth. On physical examination the GP notes evidence of breast involution and absence of axillary hair. During the consultation she mentions that she has put on weight and finds it difficult to tolerate cold weather. What is the most likely diagnosis?
   a) Cushing's syndrome
   b) Kallman's syndrome

The Complete GPVTS Stage 2 Preparation Guide: Questions and Professional Dilemmas, First Edition. Edited by Saba Khan with Neel Sharma.
© 2012 John Wiley & Sons, Ltd. Published 2012 by John Wiley & Sons, Ltd.

c) Nelson's syndrome

d) Addison's disease

e) Sheehan's syndrome

4. A 45-year-old man presents to the Emergency Department. He complains of a sudden-onset headache and visual loss. On examination you note evidence of skin pigmentation extending from the pubis to the umbilicus. He informs you that he has had surgery in the past but he is unable to recall exact details. What is the most likely diagnosis?
   a) Sheehan's syndrome
   b) Nelson's syndrome
   c) Cushing's syndrome
   d) Kallman's syndrome
   e) Addison's disease

5. A 17-year-old girl presents to her GP. She complains of problems with regards to menstruation. She also informs you that she feels her sense of smell is impaired but puts that down to a recent cold. What is the most likely diagnosis?
   a) Nelson's syndrome
   b) Cushing's syndrome
   c) Kallman's syndrome
   d) Addison's disease
   e) Sheehan's syndrome

6. A 42-year-old woman presents to her GP complaining of a gradual increase in weight. She states that she is also unable to tolerate the cold and that she feels more tired than usual. On examination you note a pulse rate of 46 beats per minute and evidence of slow relaxing reflexes. What is the most likely diagnosis?
   a) de Quervain's thryoiditis
   b) Plummer's disease
   c) Toxic multinodular goitre
   d) Hypothyroidism
   e) Graves' disease

7. A 65-year-old woman presents to her GP with a lump in her neck. The GP notes that her voice is particularly hoarse in nature. She denies any weight loss or swallowing difficulties. Blood investigations reveal an elevated serum calcitonin. What is the most likely diagnosis?
   a) Hyperthyroidism
   b) Follicular thyroid cancer
   c) Medullary cell thyroid cancer
   d) Hypothyroidism
   e) Laryngeal cancer

8. An 18-year-old girl presents to her GP. She complains of weight loss and heat intolerance. On examination you note evidence of exophthalmos and lid lag. What is the most likely diagnosis?
   a) Graves' disease
   b) De Quervain's thyroiditis
   c) Postpartum thyroiditis
   d) Thyroxine overdose
   e) None of the above

9. A 76-year-old man with type 2 diabetes is admitted to hospital with vomiting. An arterial blood gas on admission demonstrates a pH of 7.1 and potassium of 6.5 mmol/L. Past medical history includes hypertension for which he has recently been started on bendroflumethiazide. What is the most likely diagnosis?
   a) Diabetes insipidus
   b) Hypertensive crisis
   c) Hyperosmolar nonketotic state
   d) Diabetic ketoacidosis
   e) Acromegaly

10. A 27-year-old woman presents to the Emergency Department. She is a known type 1 diabetic on insulin suffering from sudden-onset abdominal pain and vomiting. On closer questioning she admits to not having taken her insulin as usual. An arterial blood gas demonstrates an elevated blood glucose and high potassium. A urine dip is positive for ketones. What is the most likely diagnosis?
    a) Hyperosmolar nonketotic state
    b) Diabetic ketoacidosis
    c) Ectopic pregnancy
    d) Diabetes insipidus
    e) None of the above

11. A 75-year-old woman is reviewed by her GP. Recent blood results demonstrate a urea of 9.9 mmol/L, a creatinine of 150 μmol/L, a sodium of 150 mmol/L, a potassium of 6.2 mmol/L and calcium of 2.01 mmol/L. Serum parathyroid hormone is elevated. What is the most likely diagnosis?
    a) Secondary hyperparathyroidism
    b) Hyperthyroidism
    c) Hypoparathyroidism
    d) Hypothyroidism
    e) Primary hyperparathyroidism

12. A 79-year-old man presents to the endocrinology outpatient clinic. He complains of gradual-onset numbness around his mouth with cramp-like pain on and off for the past two weeks. On general examination you note opposition of his thumb and flexion of the metacarpophalangeal joints. What is the most likely diagnosis?
    a) Hyperthyroidism

b) Primary hyperparathyroidism
c) Hypothyroidism
d) Secondary hyperparathyroidism
e) Hypoparathyroidism

13. A 52-year-old newly diagnosed type 2 diabetic is referred to the endocrinology outpatient department. He enquires which medication would be of most benefit to him. Background history includes congestive cardiac failure. A recent ECHO demonstrates an ejection fraction of 35%. On examination you note that he is significantly obese. What would be the most suitable treatment option?
   a) Insulin
   b) Metformin
   c) Gliclazide
   d) Diet control
   e) Pioglitazone

14. A 23-year-old woman presents to her GP. She complains of worsening acne and problems with regard to her periods. On examination you note evidence of unusual facial hair. What is the most likely diagnosis?
   a) Hypopituitarism
   b) Hyperaldosteronism
   c) Hyperprolactinaemia
   d) Hypoparathyroidism
   e) Polycystic ovary syndrome

15. A 67-year-old man presents to his GP. He complains of gradual-onset sweats, nausea and headaches over the past three weeks. On examination you note a pulse rate of 123 beats per minute and blood pressure of 195/75 mmHg. A urine dipstick demonstrates 3+ glucose. He appears notably underweight. What is the most likely diagnosis?
   a) Hypopituitarism
   b) Hyperthyroidism
   c) Phaeochromocytoma
   d) Hypoaldosteronism
   e) Hyperaldosteronism

Extended matching questions

Question 1
a) Hyperthyroidism
b) Hashimoto's thyroiditis
c) Toxic multinodular goitre
d) Thyroglossal cyst
e) Hypothyroidism
f) Simple colloid goitre
g) de Quervain's thyroiditis
h) Medullary thyroid cancer
i) Graves' disease

For each patient below, what is the most likely diagnosis?
Select ONE option only from the list above.
Each option may be selected once, more than once or not at all.

1. A 28-year-old woman presents with a lump in her neck. She denies any pain but on occasion has difficulty swallowing. On tongue protrusion you note the lump moves upwards.
2. A 47-year-old woman presents to her GP. She complains of gradual-onset weight loss and heat intolerance. On examination you note that she is in atrial fibrillation.
3. A middle-aged woman presents with a lump in her neck as well as a 2-week history of weight loss. Blood investigations demonstrate an elevated serum calcitonin.
4. A 43-year-old woman presents with pain in her neck which she describes as dull in nature. On examination you note a temperature of 39°C. Routine blood investigations demonstrate an elevated T4.
5. A 22-year-old woman presents to her GP. She complains of sudden-onset weight loss and heat intolerance. On examination you note evidence of lid lag and exophthalmos.

Question 2
a) Oral glucose tolerance test
b) Serum growth hormone
c) Urinary 5-hydroxyindoleacetic acid
d) Abdominal X-ray
e) Abdominal CT scan
f) Urinary catecholamines
g) Serum calcium
h) Thyroid function tests
i) Dexamethasone suppression test

For each patient below, what is the most likely diagnosis?
Select ONE investigative option only from the list above.
Each option may be selected once, more than once or not at all.

1. A middle-aged woman presents with new-onset headache, sweating and palpitations. She denies any loss of weight.
2. A 45-year-old man presents with new-onset headache. In addition he complains that his shoes no long fit him well. Neurological examination demonstrates evidence of a bitemporal hemianopia.
3. A 35-year-old city worker presents with sudden-onset diarrhoea and shortness of breath. On examination you note that he is flushed in appearance. He denies any recent use of antibiotics and does not smoke.
4. A 45-year-old woman presents to her GP. She complains of gradual-onset double vision and feeling faint, particularly in the morning. She comments that she has put on weight recently despite eating well and exercising regularly.
5. A 65-year-old woman presents with diarrhoea and weight loss. She denies any history of bowel cancer in the family and does not smoke. On examination you note the presence of palpable cervical lymph nodes.

Question 3

a) Hyperparathyroidism
b) Polycystic ovarian syndrome
c) Conn's syndrome
d) Phaeochromocytoma
e) Hyperaldosteronism
f) Hyperprolactinaemia
g) Diabetes insipidus
h) Acromegaly
i) Hypoparathyroidism

For each patient below, what is the most likely diagnosis?
Select ONE option only from the list above.
Each option may be selected once, more than once or not at all.

1. A middle-aged woman presents to her GP. She complains of increasing thirst and passing urine more frequently. A urine dipstick demonstrates 1+ protein. A pregnancy test is positive. On examination you note evidence of dry mucous membranes and reduced tissue turgor.
2. A 40-year-old man presents to his GP. On examination you note a prominent lower jaw and unusually large hands. During the consultation he comments that he has been sweating more frequently than usual.
3. A 33-year-old woman presents to the Emergency Department. She complains of problems with regard to her menstrual cycle. She also informs you that she has noticed her breasts are producing a milk-like substance.
4. A 46-year-old woman presents with high blood pressure. Routine blood investigations demonstrate a sodium of 155 mmol/L and a potassium of 2.8 mmol/L.
5. A 54-year-old man presents with gradual-onset headache and palpitations. Routine observations demonstrate a blood pressure of 195/45 mmHg. Blood investigations reveal an elevated plasma glucose.

Answers

Single best answer questions

Q1 b.

Addison's disease is associated with adrenocortical deficiency due to destruction of the adrenal cortex. Presenting features include myalgia, dizziness secondary to orthostatic hypotension and skin pigmentation. The latter is due to excess adrenocorticotrophic hormone (ACTH) stimulation of melanocytes. Additional symptoms may include nausea, vomiting and abdominal pain. The diagnosis is confirmed through the use of synthetic ACTH which results in minimal or no change to both aldosterone and cortisol. Steroids are the treatment of choice.

Q2 d.

Cushing's syndrome is the result of excess glucocorticoid production. Symptoms include weight gain, muscle weakness and complications such as osteoporosis, diabetes and hypertension. Diagnosis is based on measurement of urinary cortisol and the dexamethasone suppression test. The latter demonstrates an undetectable or low level of ACTH. Polymyositis is an inflammatory disorder of skeletal muscle that can also result in mobility issues such as difficulty climbing stairs and rising from a seated position. However, skin thinning and obesity are uncommon.

Q3 e.

Sheehan's syndrome occurs as a result of pituitary necrosis seen commonly as a result of bleeding during and before childbirth. Presenting features include breast involution, limited lactation and loss of axillary and pubic hair. Hypothyroidism is also common. Treatment involves the use of steroids and thyroxine.

Q4 b.

Nelson's syndrome is commonly seen after bilateral adrenalectomy for a pituitary macroadenoma. Presenting features include a headache, visual loss and skin hyperpigmentation. Serum ACTH levels are often significantly elevated in the condition. The treatment of choice includes steroids and dopamine receptor agonists such as cabergoline.

Q5 c.

Kallman's syndrome is a genetic disorder associated with GnRH deficiency. Common symptoms include incomplete puberty, decreased libido, amenorrhoea, infertility, osteoporosis and anosmia. Treatment of Kallman's syndrome involves gonadotrophin hormone replacement.

Q6 d.

Hypothyroidism in simple terms is defined as under-activity of the thyroid gland. The other causes listed above are all associated with hyperthyroidism. Common features of the former include weight gain, cold

intolerance, bradycardia, slow relaxing reflexes, myopathy and anaemia.
Treatment of choice involves the use of thyroxine replacement therapy.

Q7 c.
Medullary cell thyroid cancer is associated with mutations of the RET
oncogene. Calcitonin levels are often raised due to involvement of the
C cells. Clinical features include a hoarse voice due to recurrent laryngeal
nerve involvement and a swelling within the neck. The diagnosis relies on
fine needle aspiration, and treatment predominantly involves surgery or
radiotherapy. Follicular thyroid cancer is moderately aggressive in nature
and associated with distant metastases.

Q8 a.
Graves' disease is an autoimmune hyperthyroidism associated with thyroid
stimulating immunoglobulins and antithyroperoxidase antibodies. It can
be associated with enlargement of the thyroid gland which has an audible
bruit. Thyroid eye disease is common and features include lid lag, lid
retraction, periorbital oedema, exophthalmos, diplopia and optic nerve
compression.

Q9 c.
This is a classic presentation of hyperosmolar non-ketotic state (HONK).
It is commonly seen in patients with type 2 diabetes and presents with
profound dehydration, hyperglycaemia, vomiting, acidosis and
hyperkalaemia. It can be due to glucose overload, steroid or thiazide-based
medications. Serum osmolality is often high and treatment involves
aggressive fluid resuscitation.

Q10 b.
Diabetic ketoacidosis (DKA) is commonly seen in type 1 diabetics. It
occurs as a result of excessive catabolism secondary to insulin deficiency.
Presenting features include vomiting, polyuria, abdominal pain and in
severe cases a reduced level of consciousness. Investigative findings
demonstrate ketonuria, hyperkalaemia and metabolic acidosis.
Management comprises rehydration with saline and potassium
chloride as well as insulin.

Q11 a.
Secondary hyperparathyroidism occurs in response to the low calcium
seen typically in vitamin D deficiency or renal failure. Primary
hyperparathyroidism is typically caused by an adenoma or hyperplasia of the
gland. It is one of the most common causes of an elevated serum calcium.

Q12 e.
Hypoparathyroidism is associated with a reduction in serum calcium.
Presenting features of a lowered serum calcium include numbness around
the mouth, in addition to cramps and tetany. Physical signs of interest
include the Trousseau sign whereby carpopedal spasm is induced

following inflation of a blood pressure cuff to above systolic pressure, and the Chvostek sign whereby tapping of the facial nerve in the region of the parotid gland causes twitching of the facial muscles. Management of the low serum calcium involves the use of intravenous calcium gluconate.

Q13 b.
Metformin is particularly useful in obese type 2 diabetics as it does not cause an increase in appetite. Its main mechanism of action involves reducing glucose production and enhancing the sensitivity of the tissues to insulin. Side effects include diarrhoea and lactic acidosis. Gliclazide is a sulphonylurea which helps to promote the release of insulin. It should be avoided in overweight individuals as it results in weight gain. Pioglitazone aids in enhancing the action of insulin but is contraindicated in people with heart failure as it results in fluid retention.

Q14 e.
This is a classic presentation of polycystic ovary syndrome. Diagnostic investigations include a raised serum testosterone, raised LH to FSH ratio and an ovarian ultrasound which demonstrates evidence of multiple cysts. Antiandrogens such as cyproterone acetate are worthwhile treatments of choice.

Q15 c.
This is a rare catecholamine-producing tumour of the sympathetic nervous system. Common features include headaches, palpitations, sweating, weight loss and hypertension. To diagnose the condition one must undertake a 24-hour urine collection for metanephrines. Tumour detection is based on CT or MRI scanning. Treatment relies on surgical intervention under alpha or beta blockade.

Extended matching questions
Question 1
Q1 d.
Typical presentation of a thyroglossal cyst. It is a painless lump that is located between the thyroid isthmus and hyoid bone. Treatment is primarily surgical.

Q2 a.
Hyperthyroidism is overactivity of the thyroid gland. It is associated with weight loss, heat intolerance, palpitations, sweating and significant visual complications in the case of Graves' disease. Treatment of choice includes carbimazole, radioactive iodine or surgery.

Q3 h.
Medullary thyroid cancer is associated with an elevated serum calcitonin due to involvement of the parafollicular cells or C cells. Treatment is primarily surgical.

Q4 g.

de Quervain's thyroiditis is a transient hyperthyroidism which occurs following inflammation of the thyroid gland. Pain is common within the neck and treatment comprises aspirin or steroids.

Q5 i.

Graves disease is a common cause of hyperthyroidism. It occurs as a result of IgG antibodies directed against the TSH receptor. Eye signs which commonly occur in Graves' disease include lid lag, lid retraction, periorbital oedema, exophthalmos and diplopia. Additional features include pretibial myxoedema and onycholysis.

Question 2

Q1 f.

The diagnosis in this case is a phaeochromocytoma. Treatment of choice includes surgical resection following the use of an alpha- and beta-blocker.

Q2 a.

This patient has evidence of acromegaly. An oral glucose tolerance test is the investigation of choice and results in a lack of growth hormone suppression. Additional investigations of choice include a pituitary MRI scan.

Q3 c.

The most likely diagnosis in this case is carcinoid syndrome which comprises numerous features including facial flushing, diarrhoea and bronchospasm. Management relies on the use of somatostatin analogues, for example octreotide.

Q4 e.

The diagnosis in this case is an insulinoma. Features include hypoglycaemia partially in the mornings, diplopia, weakness and weight gain. An abdominal CT scan is the investigation of choice. Management relies on the use of surgery and diazoxide if surgery is contraindicated.

Q5 g.

The diagnosis here is most likely medullary thyroid cancer. Such cancers produce excessive levels of calcitonin which give rise to diarrhoea and an elevated serum calcium. Surgery is the treatment of choice.

Question 3

Q1 g.

Diabetes insipidus is associated with decreased production of antidiuretic hormone. Common causes include head injury, cranial surgery, hypokalaemia, pregnancy and drugs such as lithium. In severe cases desmopressin is the main form of treatment utilised. Otherwise treatment involves management of the underlying cause.

Q2 h.
Acromegaly is associated with excessive production of growth hormone commonly due to a pituitary tumour. Clinical features comprise a coarse facial appearance, enlargement of the hands and feet, hypertension, diabetes and carpal tunnel syndrome. Diagnosis is based on a failure to supress serum growth hormone with oral glucose. Treatment comprises surgical intervention, octreotide, radiotherapy or bromocriptine.

Q3 f.
Hyperprolactinaemia is associated with excess prolactin production. Causes include pregnancy, renal failure, cirrhosis, a prolactinoma and drugs such as phenothiazines and methyldopa. Dopamine agonists, for example bromocriptine, are the mainstay form of treatment.

Q4 c.
Conn's syndrome is a cause of hyperaldosteronism secondary to an aldosterone-secreting adrenal adenoma. It is associated with hypertension, hypokalaemia and a normal or high serum sodium. Treatment of choice includes surgery or the use of aldosterone antagonists, namely spironolactone.

Q5 d.
A phaeochromocytoma is a catecholamine-producing tumour of the sympathetic nervous system. Common features include headaches, palpitations, sweating and weight loss. Investigations of choice include a 24-hour collection for urinary metanephrines. Treatment is primarily surgical.

5 Gastroenterology and Nutrition

Single best answer questions

For each question below, what is the most likely answer?
Select ONE option only from the answers supplied.

1. A mother presents to the GP surgery with her 4-week-old daughter. She is concerned as her daughter has been vomiting excessively recently. On further questioning, the mother states that the vomitus is forceful in nature and occurs predominantly after feeding. Routine observations demonstrate no evidence of pyrexia, with a pulse rate within normal limits. What is the most likely diagnosis?
   a) Gastro-oesophageal reflux disease (GORD)
   b) Gastroenteritis
   c) Pyloric stenosis
   d) Urinary tract infection
   e) Posseting

2. A 32-year-old man presents to the Emergency Department with sudden-onset central abdominal pain and vomiting. He describes the pain as cramp-like and intermittent in nature with the vomitus being green in colour. Routine observations reveal a temperature of 37.6°C, blood pressure of 101/76 mmHg and pulse rate of 101 beats per minute. On examination his abdomen is notably distended with evidence of guarding. What is the most likely diagnosis?
   a) Large bowel obstruction
   b) Simple constipation
   c) Small bowel obstruction
   d) Intestinal perforation
   e) Pyloric stenosis

3. A 32-year-old man presents with sudden-onset, severe abdominal pain. He describes the pain as initially being central in origin and later

---

The Complete GPVTS Stage 2 Preparation Guide: Questions and Professional Dilemmas,
First Edition. Edited by Saba Khan with Neel Sharma.
© 2012 John Wiley & Sons, Ltd. Published 2012 by John Wiley & Sons, Ltd.

radiating to the right iliac fossa. On examination there is evidence of guarding in the right iliac fossa. What is the most likely diagnosis?
a) Incarcerated femoral hernia
b) Diverticulitis
c) Mesenteric lymphadenitis
d) Crohn's disease
e) Appendicitis

4. A 74-year-old man presents to his GP with his wife. He states that he has experienced bleeding when opening his bowels to pass motion. On further questioning he comments that he has a sense of incomplete evacuation and often strains to pass stool. His wife is particularly concerned and says that he looks thinner than normal and his clothes no longer fit him as well. What is the most likely diagnosis?
a) Rectal cancer
b) Chronic constipation
c) Diverticulitis
d) Colon cancer
e) Irritable bowel syndrome

5. An 82-year-old man presents to his GP with shortness of breath. He comments that this has been ongoing for the past few months and is associated with left-sided chest pain worse on activity and relieved by rest. He goes on to say that he also been experiencing generalised abdominal discomfort for the same duration. What is the most likely diagnosis?
a) Irritable bowel syndrome
b) Caecal cancer
c) Crohn's disease
d) Ulcerative colitis
e) Rectal cancer

6. A 35-year-old woman presents to the gastroenterology outpatient department with a 2-week history of abdominal pain and bloody diarrhoea. She is opening her bowels typically 8 times a day. On examination you note a temperature of 39°C, pulse rate of 110 beats per minute and blood pressure of 95/65 mmHg. What is the most likely diagnosis?
a) Ulcerative colitis
b) Caecal cancer
c) Crohn's disease
d) Rectal cancer
e) Irritable bowel syndrome

7. You are an F2 doctor reviewing a 28-year-old woman presenting to the gastroenterology clinic. She complains of gradual-onset generalised abdominal pain for the past 3 months. She comments that the pain improves to some degree with defecation. Her routine observations are within normal limits. On examination you note evidence of abdominal

distension but no tenderness on palpation. What is the most likely diagnosis?
a) Ulcerative colitis
b) Caecal carcinoma
c) Rectal carcinoma
d) Crohn's disease
e) Irritable bowel syndrome

8. A 54-year-old man presents to the Emergency Department with sudden-onset right upper quadrant pain and jaundice. On examination he is tachycardic at 110 beats per minute and pyrexial with a temperature of 39°C. What is the most likely diagnosis?
a) Appendicitis
b) Primary sclerosing cholangitis
c) Primary biliary cirrhosis
d) Ascending cholangitis
e) Cholecystitis

9. A 54-year-old woman presents to the Emergency Department with a 3-day history of epigastric pain radiating to her back. On examination you note evidence of central abdominal tenderness and guarding. An arterial blood gas demonstrates a pO_2 of 7.8 kPa on room air. What is the most likely diagnosis?
a) Gastro-oesophageal reflux disease
b) Cholecystitis
c) Acute pancreatitis
d) Ascending cholangitis
e) Peptic ulcer disease

10. A 53-year-old woman presents to her GP complaining of difficulty in swallowing. She comments that it came on gradually and that it affects her ability to swallow both solids and liquids. Her GP arranges a chest X-ray which demonstrates a fluid level at the aortic knuckle. What is the most likely diagnosis?
a) Gastro-oesophageal reflux disease
b) Achalasia
c) Diffuse oesophageal spasm
d) Oesophageal cancer
e) Systemic sclerosis

11. An 82-year-old man presents with progressive difficulty in swallowing. He states that he was unable to swallow solid foods initially but is now also unable to consume liquids. On examination he appears malnourished. You note during the consultation that he is coughing on occasion. What is the most likely diagnosis?
a) Diffuse oesophageal spasm
b) Gastro-oesophageal reflux disease
c) Systemic sclerosis
d) Achalasia
e) Oesophageal cancer

12. A 32-year-old woman presents to the GP with a 2-month history of rectal bleeding. She comments that the bleeding is not painful and is bright red with streaks appearing on the toilet paper. She denies any weight loss. Of note there is a family history of bowel cancer in her grandmother. What is the most likely diagnosis?
    a) Anal fissure
    b) Haemorrhoids
    c) Anal cancer
    d) Anal fistula
    e) Diverticular disease

13. A 27-year-old man presents with a 3-month history of non-bloody diarrhoea. He states that he experiences a throbbing-like perianal pain which does not really settle during the day. He denies any recent travel abroad or significant weight loss. He is a long-term smoker and drinks on occasion. On examination you note his routine observations are within normal limits. What is the most likely diagnosis?
    a) Haemorrhoids
    b) Anal fistula
    c) Anal cancer
    d) Anal fissure
    e) Diverticular disease

14. A 23-year-old man presents to his GP with a cough productive of green-coloured sputum. On examination you note evidence of yellowing of his sclerae and crepitations on chest auscultation. Routine blood investigations reveal a bilirubin of 65 μmol/L, an AST of 10 U/L, an ALT of 25 U/L and an alkaline phosphatase of 100 U/L. What is the most likely diagnosis?
    a) Primary biliary cirrhosis
    b) Primary sclerosing cholangitis
    c) Gilbert's syndrome
    d) Pancreatic cancer
    e) Budd–Chiari syndrome

15. A 32-year-old pregnant woman presents to the Emergency Department with sudden-onset abdominal pain. On examination you note evidence of jaundice, hepatomegaly and ascites. What is the most likely diagnosis?
    a) Pancreatic cancer
    b) Primary biliary cirrhosis
    c) Ascending cholangitis
    d) Budd–Chiari syndrome
    e) Gilbert's syndrome

Extended matching questions

Question 1
a) Oesophageal varices
b) Peptic ulcer disease
c) Mallory–Weiss tear
d) Gastric cancer
e) Oesophagitis
f) Zollinger–Ellison syndrome
g) Pancreatitis
h) Oesophageal cancer
i) Gastric erosions

For each patient below, what is the most likely diagnosis?
Select ONE option only from the list above.
Each option may be selected once, more than once or not at all.

1. A 32-year-old woman presents to the Emergency Department. She comments that she has been experiencing upper abdominal pain for the past few weeks. In addition she describes episodes of increased bowel frequency but without pain on defecation. She is keen to mention that she has been using Gaviscon recently, which she feels provides some partial relief. On examination you note evidence of generalised epigastric tenderness but no guarding or peritonism.
2. A 32-year-old chronic alcohol misuser presents with epigastric pain radiating to his back. On examination you note evidence of bruising around the umbilicus. Abdominal examination reveals guarding with central epigastric discomfort.
3. A 45-year-old chronic alcohol misuser presents to the Emergency Department with haematemesis. With regards to his background history you note he has been diagnosed with cirrhosis recently.
4. An 18-year-old university student presents to the Emergency Department following a drinking binge. He comments that he has been vomiting excessively and that his vomitus is bright red.
5. A 75-year-old man presents to the Emergency Department with haematemesis. He comments that he has been experiencing central abdominal pain for the past 1 month as well as weight loss of 3 kg. He states that he has also been getting full after meals more recently despite only eating moderate amounts. On examination you note evidence of a purple-coloured rash around his eyes.

Question 2
a) Stool culture
b) Urea breath test
c) Manometry
d) Colonoscopy
e) Mesenteric angiography
f) Serum ferritin

g) Transferrin saturation
h) Anti-liver kidney microsomal antibodies
i) Antinuclear antibodies

For each patient below, what is the most likely diagnosis?
Select ONE investigative option only from the list above.
Each option may be selected once, more than once or not at all.

1. A 7-year-old boy presents to the GP with jaundice and a fever. You are concerned about the possibility of autoimmune hepatitis.
2. A 75-year-old man is admitted to hospital with shortness of breath and a cough productive of green-coloured sputum. He is placed on appropriate antibiotics following evidence of consolidation on his chest X-ray. Three days later he develops diarrhoea which is non-bloody in nature.
3. A 54-year-old woman is admitted to hospital with bleeding per rectum. On examination you note evidence of an ejection systolic murmur. Abdominal examination proves unremarkable. Blood investigations demonstrate evidence of iron deficiency anaemia. She denies any weight loss and continues to experience PR bleeding.
4. A 34-year-old woman presents to her GP. She complains of an acid sensation in her mouth and minimal epigastric pain. She denies any weight loss, hematemesis or melaena. She is a non-smoker and non-drinker.
5. A 45-year-old man presents to his GP. He complains of non-specific joint discomfort and increased urinary frequency. A urine dipstick test demonstrates evidence of 3+ glucose.

Question 3
a) Biliary atresia
b) Primary biliary cirrhosis
c) Primary sclerosing cholangitis
d) Haemochromatosis
e) Alcoholic hepatitis
f) Hepatitis C
g) Budd–Chiari syndrome
h) Hepatitis B
i) Wilson disease

For each patient below, what is the most likely diagnosis?
Select ONE option only from the list above.
Each option may be selected once, more than once or not at all.

1. A 3-week-old baby girl is admitted to hospital following a routine check-up at the GP. The mother states that she has noticed her daughter's eyes are yellow and that her stools appear pale in colour. On examination you note evidence of hepatomegaly.

2. A 53-year-old man presents to his GP for a routine check-up. On examination you note an asymmetrical tremor at rest. He appears to have profound difficulty in speaking and his face appears mask-like.

3. A 38-year-old man with a background history of alcohol misuse presents to the Emergency Department. On examination you note evidence of hepatomegaly and ascites. Routine blood investigations demonstrate an abnormal liver function with an INR of 2.4.

4. A 58-year-old man presents to his GP. On examination you note evidence of a bronze discoloration of his skin. He states he feels well within himself apart from some increased desire to pass urine more frequently. A urine dipstick test demonstrates 2+ leucocytes and 4+ glucose.

5. A 38-year-old woman attends her GP complaining of generally feeling unwell. She denies any shortness of breath, cough or urinary symptoms. Routine observations are within normal limits. During the consultation you note that she is itching excessively.

Answers

Single best answer questions

Q1 c.

Pyloric stenosis is the most common cause of intestinal obstruction in infancy. It occurs due to hypertrophy of the pyloric muscular layers and may be linked to deficiency of nitric oxide synthase. It tends to occur in the first few weeks of life, commonly weeks 3 to 6. It presents as projectile vomiting after each meal, usually within 30 minutes of feeding. In some cases, the vomitus may be coffee-ground in colour due to gastritis or a Mallory–Weiss tear. On examination there may be evidence of a firm mass palpable in the right upper quadrant, often described as an 'olive' mass. GORD in children presents with recurrent regurgitation or vomiting, often with feeding difficulties and failure to thrive. Gastroenteritis would present as diarrhoea and/or vomiting. Abdominal pain is common as is a high temperature. Additional symptoms may include aching limbs. Urinary tract infections in children can present as a range of symptoms including poor feeding, failure to thrive, fever, vomiting, irritability, abdominal pain and of course urinary frequency and dysuria. Posseting is defined as the effortless, repeated regurgitation or reflux of milk after feeding. To reduce the risk of such occurrence it is advisable for babies to be given smaller, more frequent feeds and ensure that they are supported in the sitting position after feeding.

Q2 c.

Small bowel obstruction classically presents with cramp-like abdominal pain and bilious vomiting. Additional findings may include diarrhoea or constipation although the latter is often a late finding. Causes of small bowel obstruction include postsurgical adhesions, malignancy and inflammatory bowel disease. Symptoms of large bowel obstruction also include abdominal pain and vomiting but a history of constipation is more evident. Intestinal perforation presents with significant abdominal pain, guarding and peritonism. Patients are often febrile, tachycardic and hypotensive. Numerous causes exist including trauma, NSAID use, infection and malignancy. Fluid resuscitation is essential and patients should undergo immediate surgery. Pyloric stenosis is classically seen in infants and is associated with projectile vomiting.

Q3 e.

Acute appendicitis typically presents with tenderness in the periumbilical region with radiation later to the right iliac fossa. Signs of interest allied to appendicitis include the Rovsing's sign whereby individuals complain of right lower quadrant pain following palpation of the left lower quadrant, and the Dunphy sign whereby one experiences sharp pain in the right lower quadrant following coughing.

A femoral hernia results in medial thigh pain and possibly groin pain. If incarcerated, the hernia is essentially irreducible and there may be associated nausea, vomiting and symptoms of bowel obstruction. Diverticulitis presents commonly as pain in the left lower quadrant. The pain is often crampy in nature and associated with a change in bowel habit. Mesenteric lymphadenitis can mimic appendicitis. It presents with right lower quadrant pain, nausea and diarrhoea. It is however more common in children less than 15 years of age. Causative organisms include *Staphylococcus*, beta-haemolytic streptococci and *Escherichia coli*. Crohn's disease, unlike ulcerative colitis, can affect any part of the gastrointestinal tract. Symptoms include diarrhoea, abdominal pain, weight loss, fever and malaise. Small bowel Crohn's disease presents with apthous ulceration and often pain in the right iliac fossa. A mass may be palpable in this region. Colonic Crohn's disease presents with diarrhoea and associated perianal disease such as abscess formation, fistulae and skin tags.

Q4 a.
Rectal cancer presents typically with bleeding. Bowel habit change may occur but is not common. If the tumour is typically low in the rectum, individuals complain of incomplete evacuation and tenesmus, namely straining during bowel motion.

Colon cancer presents with abdominal pain, a change in bowel habit, bleeding and in severe cases evidence of intestinal obstruction. On examination there may be evidence of abdominal tenderness, a palpable mass, hepatomegaly or ascites.

Irritable bowel syndrome is a functional gastrointestinal disorder whereby there is no biochemical or structural abnormality to account for the patient's symptoms. Typical features include abdominal pain which is often relieved by defecation or associated with a change in the form of stool or bowel frequency.

Q5 b.
Caecal cancer typically presents with shortness of breath, angina and fatigue secondary to a microcytic hypochromic anaemia. Abdominal discomfort is common and a mass may be palpable. Obstructive-type symptoms do not tend to occur.

Q6 a.
Ulcerative colitis presents typically with bloody diarrhoea. Diarrhoea is common in Crohn's disease but bleeding is less likely. Severity grading in this case is high in view of her bowel frequency, temperature and the fact that she is haemodynamically unstable. Hence she would certainly require admission to hospital and a course of intravenous steroids. If after 5 to 7 days there is no improvement in her symptoms a ciclosporin infusion may be beneficial. Surgery is indicated in cases of toxic dilatation, perforation, massive haemorrhage and a failure to respond to medical treatment. Cancer is unlikely in this case in view of her age, lack of weight loss and alternating bowel habit.

Q7 e.

Irritable bowel syndrome, in accordance with the Rome III criteria, can be defined as:

- Abdominal pain or discomfort for at least 3 days per month for the past 3 months that is
- relieved by defecation
- associated with a change in the form or frequency of stool.

The condition is associated with no underlying biochemical or structural abnormality and is diagnosed often on the history alone. Unfortunately there is no cure and management is based on symptom control with the use of anti-diarrhoeal agents and dietary modification. In some cases individuals are often trialled on antidepressants such as amitriptyline as this aids in reducing bowel frequency and relieving pain. Crohn's disease and ulcerative colitis are associated with diarrhoea and abdominal pain with the latter often in conjunction with bleeding. Cancer is unlikely in this patient in view of her age and no evidence of weight loss or altered bowel habit.

Q8 d.

Ascending cholangitis presents with fever, right upper quadrant pain and jaundice, commonly known as Charcot's triad. The most likely cause of cholangitis is gallstones. Management relies on fluid resuscitation and antibiotics, typically metronidazole and ciprofloxacin. Appendicitis classically presents with periumbilical pain which radiates to the right iliac fossa. Primary sclerosing cholangitis presents with jaundice, right upper quadrant pain and itching. It is often associated with ulcerative colitis. Primary biliary cirrhosis is seen typically in women and is associated with fatigue, jaundice and malaise. Cholecystitis is associated with upper abdominal pain that radiates to the tip of the right scapula. Nausea and vomiting may also be common. Treatment of choice includes intravenous fluids, antibiotics and surgery, which is often performed laparoscopically.

Q9 c.

Pancreatitis presents with central abdominal pain. Radiation to the back is common but not always seen. The common causes of pancreatitis in the UK include alcohol and gallstones. Pancreatitis may also be seen following endoscopic retrograde cholangiopancreatography (ERCP) and the use of certain medications including steroids and azathioprine. Investigations of choice include serum amylase and lipase. Markers of severity include:

White cell count $> 15 \times 10^9$/L
Urea > 16 mmol/L
Calcium < 2 mmol/L
Albumin < 32 g/L
Glucose > 10 mmol/L
$pO_2 < 8$ kPa

AST > 200 iu/L

LDH > 600 iu/L

CRP > 150 mg/L

Symptoms of gastro-oesophageal reflux disease include heartburn, regurgitation, dysphagia and waterbrash. Peptic ulcer disease presents typically with epigastric pain. A duodenal ulcer is associated with pain at night, with gastric ulcers causing pain after meals. Vomiting is common in the latter.

Q10 b.
Achalasia is associated with progressive dysphagia allied to both solids and liquids. A fluid level on a chest X-ray is classically seen. A barium swallow reveals narrowing at the lower portion of the oesophagus. Diffuse oesophageal spasm is also associated with dysphagia for solid and liquid food as well as chest pain. A barium swallow reveals a corkscrew appearance. Oesophageal cancer presents with dysphagia, weight loss and a hoarse voice. Dysphagia is initially for solids and later liquid foods. Systemic sclerosis results in swallowing difficulties as well as other gastrointestinal manifestations including abdominal cramps and faecal incontinence.

Q11 e.
Cancer of the oesophagus presents with dysphagia initially of solid foods and later liquids. Weight loss is common and individuals may suffer a hoarse voice and cough due to involvement of the recurrent laryngeal nerve. The investigations of choice include endoscopy of the upper gastrointestinal tract as well as a barium swallow. A CT scan allows for staging and ultimately helps to govern management. Surgery is the mainstay form of treatment in those aged less than 70 with no evidence of distant spread. In this man's case, stent insertion with palliative chemotherapy or radiotherapy is likely to be the most appropriate form of treatment.

Q12 b.
Haemorrhoids are typically associated with bright red bleeding which is often noted on the toilet paper.

An anal fissure also presents with bright red bleeding but is often associated with severe pain on defecation.

Anal cancer is typically associated with a change in bowel habit, rectal bleeding and weight loss.

An anal fistula is associated with bright red bleeding as well as pain on defecation, pruritus and a mucoid discharge. Common causes include infection and inflammatory bowel disease.

Q13 b.
The most likely diagnosis here is an anal fistula occurring as a complication of Crohn's disease. Crohn's disease is commonly associated

with diarrhoea and is seen typically in smokers. Symptoms common to anal fistulae include perianal pain, pruritus and a mucoid discharge.

Q14 c.
Gilbert's syndrome is the most common cause of inherited unconjugated hyperbilirubinaemia. It arises as a result of impaired activity of glucuronyl transferase which is responsible for conjugation of bilirubin. Precipitating factors include dehydration, fasting, infection and stress. Jaundice is notable on examination and individuals may experience vague symptoms such as abdominal cramps and fatigue. Pancreatic cancer is unlikely in this case as it tends to occur in elderly individuals and is associated with painless jaundice and weight loss. Budd–Chiari syndrome is associated with obstruction to hepatic venous outflow and usually occurs in hypercoagulable states. Individuals are typically jaundiced with ascites and hepatosplenomegaly. Elevations in aminotransferases and serum alkaline phosphatase are noted.

Q15 d.
Budd–Chiari syndrome presents typically with rapidly developing symptoms of abdominal pain, hepatomegaly and ascites. It is often seen in hypercoagulable states, pregnancy, inflammatory disorders and in chronic infection. Treatment involves focusing on the underlying cause, with surgical intervention being worthwhile in the form of a shunt or liver transplant.

Extended matching questions
Question 1
Q1 f.
Zollinger–Ellison syndrome is associated with a gastrin-secreting tumour of the pancreas. It presents typically with abdominal pain and diarrhoea. Additional symptoms include heartburn and gastrointestinal bleeding. Management involves the use of proton pump inhibitors as well as surgical intervention.

Q2 g.
Pancreatitis arises commonly following long-term alcohol misuse. Epigastric pain radiating to the back is typical of the condition. Blood investigations reveal an elevated serum amylase. Management relies on the use of antibiotics, analgesia and enteral feeding to allow the pancreas to rest.

Q3 a.
Liver cirrhosis results in portal hypertension due to disruption of the vascular architecture. As a consequence, varices tend to form either within the oesophagus or stomach, which are susceptible to rupture and cause bleeding. In the UK the treatment of a variceal bleed involves the use of banding. Failing that, sclerotherapy with ethanolamine induces variceal necrosis.

Q4 c.

A Mallory–Weiss tear occurs following forceful vomiting which results typically in a tear in the gastro-oesophageal mucosal junction.

Q5 d.

Gastric cancer can present with haematemesis as well as epigastric pain and weight loss. Causative factors include smoking, a diet high in salted fish, and *Helicobacter pylori* infection. Extra manifestations include acanthosis nigricans and dermatomyositis.

Question 2

Q1 h.

Autoimmune hepatitis in children is diagnosed by the presence of anti-liver kidney microsomal antibodies. A liver biopsy is likely to show evidence of 'piecemeal' necrosis. Treatment of choice includes steroids, namely prednisolone, or other immunosuppressive agents such as azathioprine.

Q2 a.

This man is most likely to have developed *Clostridium difficile* infection following antibiotic usage. Diagnosis involves determining the presence of *C. difficile* toxin in the stool. Treatment of choice includes metronidazole or vancomycin.

Q3 e.

This presentation is consistent with angiodysplasia. It is associated with bleeding PR, iron deficiency anaemia and aortic stenosis. If a patient is actively bleeding, mesenteric angiography is the investigation of choice. Otherwise a colonoscopy is the gold standard. Treatment of choice includes argon plasma coagulation or tranexamic acid.

Q4 b.

This patient is suffering from dyspeptic-type symptoms. In accordance with NICE guidelines, patients are offered lifestyle advice initially such as diet therapies, smoking and alcohol cessation. If there is no improvement in symptoms following this, NICE advocates the use of a proton pump inhibitor or a 'test and treat' intervention using the urea breath test to exclude the presence of *Helicobacter pylori*.

Q5 g.

This man is suffering from haemochromatosis in view of his joint pains, namely chondrocalcinosis and likely diagnosis of diabetes mellitus. The gold standard investigation of choice is the transferrin saturation which is typically elevated. Serum ferritin will also be high and the total iron-binding capacity will be reduced.

Question 3

Q1 a.
Biliary atresia is associated with disturbance of the extrahepatic biliary ducts. It is seen commonly during the neonatal period. Infection and genetic factors are primary causes. In addition to pale stools one may observe dark-coloured urine. The mainstay form of treatment is surgery.

Q2 i.
Wilson's disease is a disorder of copper metabolism. It presents typically in cirrhotic individuals and can result in neuropsychiatric symptoms. On examination one may observe a greenish-brown coloured ring within the cornea known commonly as a Kayser–Fleischer ring. Blood investigations demonstrate a low serum copper and caeruloplasmin. A 24-hour urinary copper is elevated. Treatment of choice includes penicillamine, a copper chelating agent.

Q3 e.
Alcoholic hepatitis typically results in derangement of aminotransferase enzymes. The treatment is based on the use of steroids. An individual's requirement for steroids depends on their Maddrey score which is calculated based on the prothrombin time and bilirubin. A score greater than 32 necessitates steroids.

Q4 d.
This disorder is associated with excessive iron deposition within the liver as well as the heart, pancreas, pituitary and joints. It is due to a mutation of the *HFE* gene on chromosome 6. Blood investigations demonstrate an elevated serum ferritin and transferrin saturation greater than 60%. Treatment of choice includes regular venesection.

Q5 b.
Primary biliary cirrhosis is classically seen in middle-aged women. Patients are jaundiced and often experience intense itching due to excess bilirubin deposition within the skin. Serum antimitochondrial antibodies are diagnostic. Ursodeoxycholic acid has been shown to reduce disease progression.

6 Genetics

Single best answer questions

For each question below, what is the most likely answer?
Select ONE option only from the answers supplied.

1. The most likely diagnosis for a 35 year-old-man with tall stature, gynaecomastia, azoospermia and hypogonadism is:
   a) Marfan syndrome
   b) Kleinefelter syndrome
   c) Homocystinuria
   d) Beckwith–Wiedemann syndrome
   e) Vitamin-D-resistant rickets

2. The following are all recognised in Turner syndrome EXCEPT:
   a) There is an increased risk of hypertension
   b) The patient is of short stature
   c) Bicuspid aortic valve
   d) Short fourth metacarpals
   e) 50% chance of future offspring inheriting the disease

3. The following diseases are inherited in an autosomal dominant manner EXCEPT:
   a) Adult polycystic kidney disease
   b) Huntington chorea
   c) Achondroplasia
   d) Wilson disease
   e) Myotonic dystrophy

4. Trisomy 21 may be associated with:
   a) Endocardial cushion defect (atrioventricular septal defect)
   b) Tricuspid atresia
   c) Transposition of the great arteries
   d) Aortic stenosis
   e) Coarctation of the aorta

The Complete GPVTS Stage 2 Preparation Guide: Questions and Professional Dilemmas,
First Edition. Edited by Saba Khan with Neel Sharma.
© 2012 John Wiley & Sons, Ltd. Published 2012 by John Wiley & Sons, Ltd.

5. A 35-year-old woman presents with calf swelling. Ultrasound studies confirm a deep vein thrombosis (DVT). The most likely cause is:
   a) Antithrombin III deficiency
   b) Factor V Leiden
   c) Lupus anticoagulant
   d) Protein C deficiency
   e) Protein S deficiency

6. Breast cancer is more likely in patients with mutations in one of the two susceptibility genes, *BRCA1* and *BRCA2*.
   Which two of the following statements are correct with reference to these gene mutations?
   a) Patients with these gene mutations have over a 60% chance of developing breast cancer.
   b) Patients with this gene mutation have over a 60% chance of developing ovarian cancer.
   c) Gene mutations in these genes account for 50% of all breast cancers.
   d) Patients with these gene mutations have a 30% chance of developing ovarian cancer.
   e) The *BRCA* gene mutation is classified as one of the major risk factors for breast cancer.

7. A healthy, recently married 25-year-old patient presents to your surgery. His younger sibling is known to have infantile polycystic kidney disease. Both of his parents are not known to have any chronic illness. What is the chance of him being a carrier?
   a) 1 in 4 (25%)
   b) 1 in 3 (33%)
   c) 1 in 2 (50%)
   d) 2 in 3 (66%)
   e) 1 in 1 (100%)

8. The following are all true with regard to autosomal dominant polycystic kidney disease (ADPKD) EXCEPT:
   a) The kidneys are often enlarged
   b) Treatment of blood pressure is important to prevent cardiovascular disease
   c) Is associated with hepatic fibrosis
   d) Cysts arise from nephrons and collecting tubules
   e) Patients may have associated hepatic cysts

9. A 7-year-old with homozygous sickle cell anaemia presents to the Emergency Department complaining of chest pain. He has a temperature of 38.3°C, blood pressure 90/65 mmHg, tachycardic with a white cell count of 15×10^9/L. You speak to his parents and they inform you they have recently emigrated from West Africa. They are unsure of their child's vaccination history and have never given him prophylactic antibiotics. Which of the following is the most likely cause?

a) *Staphylococcus* aureus septicaemia
b) Vancomycin-resistant enterococcus septicaemia
c) Salmonella septicaemia
d) Mycoplasma pneumoniae septicaemia
e) Streptococcus pneumoniae septicaemia

10. A 40-year-old man is brought to your clinic by his concerned family. He appears more 'fidgety' than usual, has become increasing forgetful and aggressive. His parents divorced early but his wife tells you his father had similar problems and died at the age of 55. What is the most likely diagnosis?
a) Pick disease
b) Alzheimer disease
c) Senile chorea
d) Wilson disease
e) Huntington disease

11. Which of the following is CORRECT regarding the mode of inheritance of mitochondrial disorders?
a) Are only transmitted maternally
b) Are only transmitted paternally
c) Autosomal dominant
d) Autosomal recessive
e) X-linked

12. A 25-year-old man presents to your surgery having noticed a new 'yellow tinge' to his eyes. He denies excess alcohol consumption or illicit drug use and is otherwise well. The only abnormal blood test result reveals a mildly elevated bilirubin. What is the most likely diagnosis?
a) Primary biliary cirrhosis
b) Dubin–Johnson syndrome
c) Gilbert syndrome
d) Primary sclerosing cholangitis
e) Hepatitis C

13. A 14-year-old child is brought to your surgery by his concerned mother. He complains of a difficulty seeing the whiteboard at school and his mother has noticed large brown 'spots' on his body. On testing his visual acuity, you find a focal area of reduced acuity, with preserved vision elsewhere. What is the most likely diagnosis?
a) Neurofibromatosis type I (NF1)
b) Neurofibromatosis type II (NF2)
c) Tuberous sclerosis
d) Turcot syndrome
e) von Hippel–Lindau disease

14. Which of the following could NOT be a possible source of DNA?
    a) Red blood cell
    b) Skin cell
    c) Liver cell
    d) Brain cell
    e) Kidney cell

15. You discover that a patient being investigated for liver disease has confirmed haemochromatosis. A liver biopsy excludes underlying cirrhosis. You recall the patient to your clinic, where he asks you how the disease is treated. You inform him that the mainstay of treatment is:
    a) Transfusion
    b) Chelation
    c) Phlebotomy
    d) Iron supplements
    e) Liver transplantation

Extended matching questions

Question 1
For each of the following scenarios select the SINGLE best answer from the list below:
a) Factor VII
b) Autosomal dominant
c) Autosomal recessive
d) Protein C
e) Factor VIII
f) Epiphysis overgrowth
g) Diaphysis overgrowth
h) Metaphysis overgrowth
i) Mitochondrial
j) X-linked
k) Factor IX
l) Factor X
m) Kallikrein

1. A young boy is brought to your surgery with easy bruising following trivial injury. After sending him for testing, you discover he has haemophilia A. Of the above, which is the most likely to be deficient?
2. The parents of the child learn the disease has a genetic element. Which of the options above is the correct mode of inheritance?
3. Of the above, which is the most likely radiological manifestation?

Question 2
For each of the following scenarios select the SINGLE best answer from the list below:
a) Gaucher disease
b) Maple syrup urine disease
c) Phenylketonuria
d) Homocystinuria
e) Achondroplasia
f) Prader–Willi syndrome
g) Familial short stature
h) Alkaptonuria
i) Constitutional delay
j) Acromegaly
k) Hyperthyroidism
l) Turner syndrome
m) Diabetes

1. A heel-prick blood sample is sent for analysis as part of the newborn screening testing for inborn errors of metabolism. Of the above, what is routinely tested for?

2. A 10-year-old boy is brought to your surgery by his concerned mother. He is of short stature, morbidly obese and requires extensive educational support. On examination, you note he has small hands and feet. What is the most likely diagnosis?

3. A child with a known genetic abnormality is brought to your surgery. He is of short stature with megalencephaly (large head) and frontal bossing. You also note there is disproportionate shortening of the limbs with a normal trunk length. What is the likely diagnosis?

Question 3

For each of the following questions select the SINGLE best answer from the list below:

a) Chromosome 21
b) Chronic myelogenous leukaemia (CML)
c) Chronic lymphocytic leukaemia (CLL)
d) Chromosome 13
e) Chromosome 17
f) Hodgkin lymphoma
g) Non-Hodgkin lymphoma
h) Chromosome 18
i) Burkitt lymphoma
j) Primary cerebral lymphoma
k) Lymphoma (HIV-related)
l) Chromosome 16
m) Small bowel lymphoma

1. Patau syndrome is associated with a trisomy of which chromosome?
2. The Philadelphia chromosome is a characteristic chromosomal abnormality associated with which haematological condition?
3. A 28-year-old patient presents with fever, night sweats and weight loss; he has focal lymphadenopathy. What is the most likely diagnosis?

Answers

Single best answer questions

Q1 b.

Kleinefelter syndrome is a chromosomal disorder (47XXY) which affects 1 in 1,000 males. The combination of tall stature, gynaecomastia, azoospermia and hypogonadism is considered diagnostic; however, confirmation can be achieved by chromosomal analysis. The condition involves the loss of both Leydig cells and seminiferous tubular dysgenesis. Other features include sparse facial hair, atrophic testes and mild learning difficulties. Marfan syndrome, homocystinuria and Beckwith–Wiedemann syndrome can all result in tall stature but the remaining features described are not characteristic of these conditions.

Q2 e.

Turner syndrome is a sex chromosome monosomy in which the individual has a single X chromosome without a second X or Y chromosome (45X0). The condition is associated with characteristic physical abnormalities such as short stature, webbed neck, shield chest with widely spaced nipples, short fourth metacarpals, low hairline and lymphoedema. It has an incidence of approximately 1 in 2,500. The main abnormality is gonadal dysgenesis, the consequences of which are primary amenorrhoea and infertility. Up to 15% will have a bicuspid aortic valve. The risk of hypertension is increased due to essential hypertension, renal abnormalities and coarctation of the aorta (5–10%).

Q3 d.

Wilson disease is an autosomal recessive disorder with a molecular defect within a copper-transporting ATPase encoded by a gene (*ATP7B*) located on chromosome 13. The inborn error of copper metabolism results in copper deposition in a multitude of organs, including the liver, basal ganglia and cornea (Kayser–Fleischer ring). As a consequence, the disease may manifest with neurological and psychiatric symptoms, or liver disease.

Q4 a.

Trisomy 21 (Down syndrome) is seen in approximately 1 in 800 live births. Endocardial cushion defects are the most commonly encountered congenital cardiac defect (~40%). Other recognised structural abnormalities include ventricular septal defect (VSD), secundum atrial septal defect (ASD), tetralogy of Fallot, patent ductus arteriosus (PDA) and pulmonic stenosis.

Q5 b.

Factor V Leiden is an autosomal dominant condition which exhibits incomplete dominance and results in a factor V variant which cannot be as easily degraded by aPC (activated Protein C). It is the most common hereditary hypercoagulability disorder among Eurasians (3–5% of the

Western population) and is thought to increase the risk of venous thrombosis by 3–8-fold for heterozygous individuals and 30–140-fold for homozygous individuals. The abnormal gene is found in 30% of patients with recurrent venous thrombosis.

Q6 a, d.
The *BRCA* gene mutation accounts for 2–3% of all breast cancers, and increases susceptibility to breast and ovarian cancer. The major risk factors for breast cancer are gender, age, lack of breast feeding and childbearing, higher hormone levels, and socioeconomic status. Other factors such as alcohol intake and smoking as well as family history, gene mutation and fibrocystic breast changes are also contributing risk factors.

Q7 d.
Infantile polycystic kidney disease is an autosomal recessive condition. Those affected by the disease will have mutations in both alleles of the gene. We know both parents are well, therefore the chances of their offspring being affected by the disease is 1 in 4 (25%), with a 1 in 2 (50%) chance of being a carrier and 1 in 4 (25%) chance of being neither affected nor a carrier. In this particular case, we know the patient is healthy and therefore unaffected by the disease. We can therefore remove the 1 in 4 (25%) chance that the patient is affected by the disease. This leaves a 2 in 3 (66%) chance of him being a carrier and a 1 in 3 (33%) chance of him not being a carrier.

Q8 c.
ADPKD affects approximately 1 in 1,000 people. In 90% of patients, the affected gene is located on chromosome arm 16p. The disease is characterised by the presence of renal cysts and it is thought that 54% of cysts will appear by the first decade of life, 72% by the second decade and 86% by the third decade. As the size of cysts increase, the kidneys enlarge and may lose their reniform shape. Cysts can also be found in the liver, pancreas and spleen. There is also a known association with intracranial berry aneurysms and mitral valve prolapse. Adequate blood pressure management and monitoring of renal function +/− need for renal replacement therapy are the predominant clinical concerns. Hepatic fibrosis is known to occur in patients with autosomal recessive polycystic kidney disease (ARPKD).

Q9 e.
Patients with sickle cell disease are functionally hyposplenic in the first few years of life and become anatomically asplenic (due to splenic infarction/ atrophy) by the second decade of life. Absent or defective splenic function is associated with a high risk of bacterial septicaemia with encapsulated organisms such as *Streptococcus pneumoniae*, *Haemophilus influenzae*, *Nesseria meningitides* and *Chlamydia trachomatis*. Infections secondary to these organisms are the most common to occur in patients with sickle cell disease. Appropriate vaccination and prophylactic antibiotics are the main strategies adopted in trying to prevent this disease complication.

Children with sickle cell disease are also more susceptible to salmonella infections which are usually limited to the gastrointestinal tract. Children with sickle cell disease, however, are more prone than other children to develop serious invasive salmonella infections of the bone (osteomyelitis), as well as sepsis and meningitis.

Q10 e.

Huntington disease (HD) is an incurable, adult-onset, autosomal dominant inherited disorder associated with cell loss within a specific subset of neurons in the basal ganglia and cortex. The disease is characterised clinically by disorders of movement (mild chorea may pass for fidgetiness), progressive dementia, and psychiatric and/or behavioural disturbance. The condition is usually clinically apparent by the third or fourth decade and is caused by the expansion of a CAG triplet repeat in the HD gene on 4p16.

Patients with Alzheimer disease usually have a slowly progressive dementia and belong to an older age group. Senile chorea is a rare disorder beginning in persons older than 60 years; the disordered movements are usually less prominent than in patients with HD. Pick disease affects the frontal and temporal lobes. Clinically, it resembles HD; however, the age of onset is usually later in life and with a different underlying pathology.

Q11 a.

Mitochondrial disorders are caused by mutations in the mitochondrial genome. Almost all mitochondrial DNA molecules are inherited from the oocyte, therefore all associated diseases can only be maternally transmitted.

Q12 c.

Gilbert syndrome is the most common inherited cause of unconjugated hyperbilirubinaemia. This autosomal recessive condition is characterised by intermittent jaundice in the absence of haemolysis or underlying liver disease. The rise in bilirubin levels is almost always mild. The condition can be precipitated in periods of stress, with prevalence thought to be 3–7% of the population.

Q13 a.

Neurofibromatosis (NF) is a multisystem genetic disorder caused by a mutation or deletion of the NF1 gene. It is commonly associated with cutaneous, neurological and orthopaedic manifestations. The most recognisable clinical feature of NF1 is the appearance of brown café-au-lait spots; these occur in 95% of NF1 patients and are frequently the first manifestation of the disorder. Tuberous scleroses, NF2, von Hippel–Lindau and Turcot syndrome are not associated with café-au-lait spots. Optic gliomas also are a frequent manifestation, with a 25% incidence in NF1 patients. Other clinical criteria of NF1 include: freckling in the axillary region; neurofibromas (≥ 2 or 1 plexiform); two or more Lisch nodules; an osseous lesion or thinning of the long bone cortex with or without pseudoarthritis; and a first-degree relative with NF1.

Q14 a.
Red blood cells do not contain nuclei or DNA; all the other mentioned cells could be a source of DNA.

Q15 c.
Haemochromatosis leads to an abnormal accumulation of iron in parenchymal organs, which can progress to eventual organ toxicity. It is the most common inherited liver disease in white people and the most prevalent autosomal recessive genetic disorder. The gene is linked to the short arm of chromosome 6.

The aim of treatment is to remove the excess iron before it can lead to irreversible organ damage, with phlebotomy serving this purpose. Iron supplements should be avoided. Liver transplantation is the only feasible option if the patient progresses to end-stage liver disease despite iron-reduction therapy.

Extended matching questions
Question 1
Q1 e.
Haemophilia is the oldest known bleeding disorder. The deficiency or absence of factor VIII leads to haemophilia A.

Q2 j.
It is a disease that affects males with the defective gene found on the X chromosome.

Q3 f.
Approximately 50% of patients with haemophilia develop permanent changes in the joint. Appearances include: joint haemorrhage/joint effusion; osteoporosis; erosions; bone cysts; articular cartilage destruction; overgrowth of the epiphysis; and degenerative arthritis.

Question 2
Q1 c.
Heel-prick sampling is part of the routine neonatal screening and should be performed on all neonates by 5–8 days of age. Other conditions tested for include congenital hypothyroidism, sickle cell disease and thalassaemia, cystic fibrosis and medium-chain acyl CoA dehydrogenase.

Q2 f.
Prader–Willi syndrome (PWS) is a disorder caused by a deletion or disruption of chromosome 15. Other features of the disease include hypotonia, hypogonadotrophic hypogonadism and strabismus. Characteristic facial features include narrow bifrontal diameter, narrow nasal bridge and downturned mouth.

Q3 f.
Achondroplasia is inherited as an autosomal dominant trait and is the most common inherited short-limb dwarfism. The frequency of the disease is thought to range from 1 case per 15,000–40,000 births. Other salient features of the condition include a midface hypoplasia, lumbar lordosis, genu varum and a trident hand configuration.

Question 3
Q1 d.
Patau syndrome occurs in 1/25,000 births. Individuals with the disease suffer from mental retardation, microcephaly, cleft lip and palate, postaxial polydactyly, abnormal brain development (arrhinencephaly, holoprosencephaly), cardiac dextroposition and ventricular septal defect. Prognosis is usually poor with survival beyond 6 months very rare.

Q2 b.
The Philadelphia chromosome is associated with CML and is present in the bone marrow cells of sufferers in 95% of the cases. It is usually due to a reciprocal translocation between the long arms of chromosome 22 and 9. The presence of the Philadelphia (Ph) chromosome is not sufficiently specific to diagnose CML, since it is also found in acute lymphoblastic leukaemia (ALL, 25–30% in adult and 2–10% in paediatric cases) and occasionally in acute myelogenous leukaemia (AML).

Q3 f.
The most likely diagnosis is Hodgkin lymphoma, the constellation of fever, night sweats and weight loss are known as B symptoms. Patients can also describe generalised pruritis. Clinical examination can reveal focal lymphadenopathy and also hepatosplenomegaly if there is more extensive tumour infiltration.

7 Haematology

For each question below, what is the most likely answer?
Select one or more options from the answers supplied.

1. Which of the following is a NOT a cause of macrocytic anaemia?
   a) Phenytoin
   b) Alcohol excess
   c) Hyperthyroidism
   d) Myelodysplastic syndrome
   e) Vitamin B12/folate deficiency

2. Erythropoietin is a treatment for which two types of anaemia of chronic disease?
   a) Tuberculosis
   b) Renal failure
   c) Rheumatoid arthritis
   d) Malignancy
   e) Systemic vasculitis

3. Which one of the following leads only to neutropenia?
   a) Severe sepsis
   b) Viral infections
   c) Metastatic disease
   d) Burns
   e) Myocardial infarction

4. Which condition features eosinophilia?
   a) Parasitic infection
   b) Cushing syndrome
   c) Pulmonary embolism
   d) Drug treatment with antihistamines
   e) Iron deficiency

The Complete GPVTS Stage 2 Preparation Guide: Questions and Professional Dilemmas,
First Edition. Edited by Saba Khan with Neel Sharma.
© 2012 John Wiley & Sons, Ltd. Published 2012 by John Wiley & Sons, Ltd.

5. Pernicious anaemia is best related to which single statement?
a) Higher incidence in blood group B
b) Usually diagnosed by the age of 40
c) Found equally in females and males
d) Incidence is 1 in 100,000
e) Three times increased risk of gastric carcinoma

6. Iron absorption from the gut is aided by which one of the following?
a) Coffee
b) Tea
c) Red wine
d) Tofu
e) Orange juice

7. Which one of the following statements is correct with regard to haemophilia A?
a) Factor VII deficiency
b) Inherited in an X-linked dominant pattern
c) Found equally in females and males
d) Incidence is 1 in 1,000 births
e) There is a high rate of new mutations – 30% have no family history

8. Which statement about anticoagulation with warfarin is correct?
a) Is safe for use in pregnancy
b) Has a narrow therapeutic range
c) Protamine sulfate reverses the effects of warfarin
d) Anticoagulation should be lifelong after a pulmonary embolus
e) Has been replaced with new direct thrombin inhibitors, e.g. dabigatran, as it does not require monitoring

9. Low molecular weight heparin (LMWH) is NOT suitable for use in which one of the following situations?
a) Recent neurosurgery
b) During pregnancy
c) Concurrent treatment with warfarin
d) Use with prosthetic heart valves
e) Postoperative prevention of DVT/PE

10. When considering myeloma, which is the correct statement?
a) The diagnosis requires a positive test for Bence-Jones protein
b) Male to female incidence is 4:1
c) Peak age of incidence is 85
d) Produces a monoclonal band or paraprotein on serum electrophoresis
e) Has an excellent prognosis for most patients

11. Following a splenectomy which TWO infections present the higher risk?

a) *Clostridium difficile*
b) *Neisseria meningitidis*
c) Varicella zoster
d) *Streptoccocus pneumoniae*
e) *Pseudomonas aeruginosa*

12. Which two of the following are found in vitamin B12 and folate deficiency but not in iron deficiency?
    a) Splenomegaly
    b) Increased risk of infections
    c) Peripheral neuropathy
    d) Glossitis and angular stomatitis
    e) Spoon-shaped nails (koilonychias)

13. Which one of the following findings are NOT found on the blood film of a patient with a haemolytic anaemia?
    a) Spherocytes
    b) Schistocytes
    c) Sickle cells
    d) Hypochromic microcytic anaemia
    e) Thrombocytopenia

14. In an emergency scenario, which blood group is the universal donor?
    a) Group A Rh positive
    b) Group O Rh negative
    c) Group AB Rh negative
    d) Group B Rh positive
    e) Group O Rh positive

15. Which of the following would make a diagnosis of Hodgkin lymphoma rather than non-Hodgkin lymphoma?
    a) Night sweats
    b) Superficial lymphadenopathy
    c) Weight loss
    d) Fever
    e) Reed-Sternberg cells

Extended matching questions

Question 1
Select one or more options from the list for the following questions:
a) Bone marrow failure
b) Anaemia of chronic disease
c) Renal failure
d) Haemolysis
e) Hypothyroidism
f) Immunosuppressive cytotoxic therapy
g) Alcoholism
h) Cocaine abuse
i) Hyperthyroidism
j) Severe acute haemorrhage
k) Phenytoin therapy
l) Thalassaemia
m) Blood transfusion
n) Iron therapy
o) Exchange transfusion
p) Conservative management

1. A patient presents with a blood film showing macrocytes, and blood results with a raised MCV, raised gamma GT and raised ALT. Which one of the above is the most likely diagnosis?
2. A 43-year-old man with a known history of metastatic cancer has previously been treated with chemotherapy but he is now to receive palliative care. His blood film shows hypochromic normocytic cells. His blood results show Hb 8 g/dL. What is the most likely diagnosis and what is the best treatment?
3. A patient presents with symptoms of feeling cold, with dry skin and weight gain. Her blood film and results show a macrocytic anaemia. What is the most likely diagnosis?

Question 2
Pick one of the following options in answer to each question below:
a) African heritage
b) Asian heritage
c) Deoxygenated
d) Oxygenated
e) Haemolysis
f) Sickling
g) Fragmentation
h) Autosomal recessive
i) Autosomal dominant
j) Mosaicism
k) Sickle cell anaemia
l) Sickle cell trait

m) Vaso-occlusive crisis
n) Aplastic crisis
o) Splenic sequestration crisis

1. In which ethnic group is sickle cell disease most commonly found, and what is the genetic inheritance of the condition?
2. A 14-year-old boy of African origin presents with his father. He has recently been advised by another doctor that he is a sickle cell 'carrier'. He would like to know what this means and also what would happen to his blood cells if he becomes unwell.
3. A 24-year-old man with known sickle cell disease presents looking pale and tired. On examination he is pale and tachycardic. What is the most likely diagnosis?

Question 3
Pick one or more from the following list in answer to the questions below:
a) Anisocytosis
b) Poikilocytosis
c) Acanthocytes
d) Target cells
e) Macrocytosis
f) Microcytosis
g) Rouleaux
h) Schistocytes
i) Hypochromasia
j) Polychromasia
k) Reticulocytes
l) Malarial parasites
m) Toxic granulation
n) Hairy cells

1. A patient with inflammatory bowel disease and anaemia presents to the GP for a blood test and blood film. The blood film shows red blood cells as though they are 'stacks of coins'. What is the correct term for this finding?
2. An 85-year-old man has had a mechanical heart valve for almost 10 years. What abnormality might you expect to see on a blood film?
3. A 34-year-old woman has rheumatoid arthritis, diagnosed at age 20. What change might you expect to see on a blood film?

Answers

Single best answer questions

Q1 c.
The common causes that are not listed above include haemolysis leading to reticulocytosis, cytotoxic drugs and hypothyroidism.

Q2 b, d.
The treatment for anaemia of chronic disease focuses on treatment of the underlying disorder. In renal failure this is partly due to erythropoietin deficiency, so replacement therapy is effective, and can also be used to treat symptomatic anaemia in malignancy.

Q3 b.
Bacterial infection usually leads to neutrophilia, however in severe sepsis neutropenia can be found. Metastatic disease can produce neutrophilia, but neutropenia is found in the presence of bone marrow failure. Trauma, including burns, leads to neutrophilia, as can inflammation from a myocardial infarction.

Q4 a.
Asthma and allergic conditions, along with parasitic infections, are the commonest causes. Addison disease, malignancy and many types of skin disease (eczema, urticaria, pemphigus) feature eosinophilia. Antihistamines are commonly used to treat allergy, but penicillins can cause a raised eosinophil count.

Q5 e.
Pernicious anaemia is found usually over the age of 60, with a female to male ratio of 3:2. Incidence is 1 in 1000, and found more commonly in people with blood group A. It is reported to lead to a three times increased risk of gastric carcinoma.

Q6 e.
A number of dietary factors influence iron absorption. Ascorbic acid and citrate increase iron uptake in the duodenum. Conversely, iron absorption is inhibited by plant phytates and tannins. These compounds also chelate iron, but prevent its uptake. Phytates are prominent in wheat and some other cereals, while tannins are prevalent in (non-herbal) teas. Beverages such as red wine, coffee, black tea, herbal teas and cocoa are rich in polyphenols, which lower the absorption of iron from foods. Soy contains iron that is easily absorbed; however, a compound found in soy products such as tofu inhibits the body's ability to absorb iron.

Q7 e.
Haemophilia A is due to a factor VIII deficiency caused by an X-linked recessive disorder, in 1 in 10,000 male births, but there is a high rate of new mutations – 30% have no family history.

Q8 b.

Warfarin treatment has a narrow therapeutic range, which varies according to the condition being treated, hence regular monitoring is needed. It is contraindicated in pregnancy, peptic ulcer disease, bleeding disorders and severe hypertension. Heparin is reversed with protamine sulfate; vitamin K reverses warfarin. After a first pulmonary embolus, treatment is for at least three months' duration if low risk and without permanent risk factors.

Q9 a.

LMWH has become the preferred management for prevention and treatment of venous thromboembolism and in acute coronary syndrome. It is initiated in the acute setting and continues until warfarin levels are therapeutic where longer-term anticoagulation is intended, and then can be stopped. It is even used in pregnancy where indicated, as warfarin is contraindicated. LMWH is contraindicated in bleeding disorders, peptic ulcer disease, post neurosurgery and cerebral haemorrhage.

Q10 d.

Myeloma is a malignant neoplasm of plasma cells that arises in the bone marrow. Presentation is with anaemia, bone pain, skeletal destruction, pathological fractures, or Bence-Jones protein found in the urine in 2/3 of cases. Peak age is 70 with 1:1 male to female ratio. A single clone of identical immunoglobulin produces a monoclonal band or para protein on serum or urine electrophoresis. Median survival is 3 years.

Q11 b, d.

Asplenic patients are at risk of overwhelming infection, most often by encapsulated bacteria such as *Streptococcus pneumoniae, Salmonella typhi, Neisseria meningitidis, E. coli, Hemophilus influenzae* and *Klebsiella pneumoniae*. The risk is greater in the early months and years following splenectomy.

Q12 a, c.

Vitamin B12, folate and iron deficiency can lead to increased risk of infections, glossitis and angular stomatitis, while koilonychia is a feature of iron deficiency. Splenomegaly and peripheral neuropathy are features of vitamin B12 deficiency.

Q13 e.

Spherocytes are found in hereditary spherocytosis, schistocytes in microangiopathic haemolytic anaemia, sickle cells in sickle cell anaemia, and a hypochromic microcytic picture is seen with thalassaemia. Thrombocytopenia would suggest an alternate diagnosis if found alone.

Q14 b.

Where possible, especially prior to major surgery, a 'group and save' is done so the patient's blood group and rhesus status are known in advance.

This allows blood to be cross-matched with the donor blood prior to transfusion. However, in the emergency setting blood group O Rh negative can be used.

Q15 e.
Both Hodgkin lymphoma and non-Hodgkin lymphoma are types of cancer that originate from lymphocytes. The presenting symptoms can be very similar, though fever, night sweats and weight loss are less common in non-Hodgkin than in Hodgkin and would suggest disseminated disease.

The main difference between Hodgkin and non-Hodgkin lymphoma is in the specific lymphocyte each involves. If there is the presence of the specific abnormal Reed-Sternberg cell, the lymphoma is classified as Hodgkin. If the Reed-Sternberg cell is not present, the lymphoma is classified as non-Hodgkin. The distinction is important because the treatment for each type can be very different.

Extended matching questions
Question 1
Q1 g.
Alcohol abuse leads to folate deficiency and therefore a macrocytic picture on blood film. The raised gamma GT and ALT also indicate liver disease.

Q2 b, p.
This patient has anaemia of chronic disease secondary to his malignancy. The Hb of 8 g/dL, though low, is likely to be compensated and hence conservative management is appropriate.

Q3 e.
The patient has hypothyroidism which causes a raised MCV, however a normocytic anaemia can also be present.

Question 2
Q1 a, h.
The condition is inherited in an autosomal recessive condition and some three-quarters of sickle cell cases are believed to occur in Africa.

Q2 f, l.
The patient has sickle cell trait which means he carries one sickle cell gene with one normal gene. He would essentially remain asymptomatic, with caution required when undergoing general anaesthetic risk and in situations of hypoxic insult.

Q3 n.
This occurs in patients with sickle cell disease as a result of parvovirus B19. This virus attacks red cell production and is normally self-limiting.

However, in patients with sickle cell disease, the rapid red cell turnover results in acute severe loss of red blood cell volume. These patients often need acute blood transfusions to help them recover.

Question 3

Q1 g.
Rouleaux. This is seen in inflammatory conditions, anaemia, multiple myeloma and macroglobulinaemia.

Q2 h.
Schistocytes are fragmented red blood cells that have been damaged. Other conditions that cause fragility of red blood cells also result in this finding.

Q3 f.
Microcytosis, or small red blood cells, are also seen typically in iron deficiency anaemia, chronic disease and thalassaemia.

8 Immunology

For each question below, what is the most likely answer?
Select ONE option only from the answers supplied.

1. You are an F2 doctor in general practice. It is a Friday afternoon and you are just about to leave when the receptionist transfers a call from the local laboratory. The pathologist states that Miss M, 28 years old, has an abnormal blood film with the presence of blast cells. What do you do?
   a) Leave the result for the requesting doctor to deal with on Monday. Patient continuity is important.
   b) Look through her notes. She attended the previous week with tiredness and bruises but is otherwise well. You decide to call her first thing on Monday to inform her that she will be referred to a haematologist.
   c) Call her to arrange a home visit that evening.
   d) Call the out-of-hours provider to arrange a home visit for that evening if she deteriorates.
   e) Call the patient and inform her that she needs to be seen in hospital immediately.

2. You are an F2 doctor in general practice. You see a mother with her 5-year-old son. He presents with 'yet another infection'. From his notes, he has attended at least 10 times with recurrent infections needing antibiotics in the last 6 months. You diagnose an upper respiratory chest infection. What is your management?
   a) Explain that infections are common in this age group, especially when starting nursery, and reassure his mother.
   b) Perform a full examination and prescribe antibiotics.
   c) Refer to a paediatrician.
   d) Consider an immunological cause and send him for some blood tests.
   e) Advise conservative management, explaining that repeated antibiotic courses may lead to resistance.

The Complete GPVTS Stage 2 Preparation Guide: Questions and Professional Dilemmas,
First Edition. Edited by Saba Khan with Neel Sharma.
© 2012 John Wiley & Sons, Ltd. Published 2012 by John Wiley & Sons, Ltd.

3. Which of the following concerning B-cell deficiency is correct?
   a) It includes selective IgA deficiency
   b) It is usually linked with infections caused by Gram-positive organisms
   c) The patient may be completely asymptomatic
   d) May not require any treatment
   e) All of the above

4. Which of the following indicates testing for serum immunoglobulins?
   a) Suspected myeloma
   b) Liver disease
   c) Diagnosis of sarcoidosis
   d) Suspected immunodeficiency
   e) All of the above

5. You are an F2 doctor working in general practice. A 30-year-old woman comes to see you with a 3-month history of severe hand erythema and dryness. She has no history of atopy or eczema. Her symptoms improved when on holiday. She has recently started work as a laboratory assistant. What is your differential diagnosis and management?
   a) Atopic dermatitis: emollients
   b) Occupational dermatitis: refer to a dermatologist
   c) Skin infection: prescribe Trimovate
   d) Occupational allergy: refer to allergy clinic
   e) Eczema: emollients and steroids

6. You are working in the Emergency Department. A 4-year-old boy is brought in having been stung by a bee. His mother found him in the playground unconscious. He recovered on being administered adrenaline. Which of the following mediated this response?
   a) IgA
   b) IgE
   c) IgM
   d) IgG
   e) All of the above

7. You are an F2 doctor working in general practice. You see a 17-year-old girl for a review after she was admitted to the Emergency Department with angioedema. There was no urticaria and she has now fully recovered. Her mother states that she also suffers from a similar condition. What is the most useful test?
   a) IgE
   b) C3
   c) C4
   d) C1 esterase inhibitor
   e) Full blood count

8. A 30-year-old female has a history of repeated sinus and lower respiratory tract infections. She has been told she has a specific immunoglobulin deficiency. Which immunoglobulin is most likely deficient?
   a) IgD
   b) IgA
   c) IgE
   d) IgG
   e) IgM

9. Which one of the following is NOT increased as part of the acute phase response?
   a) Serum amyloid A
   b) C-reactive protein (CRP)
   c) Ferritin
   d) Ceruloplasmin
   e) Albumin

10. Which one of the following cell types is phagocytic?
    a) Lymphocyte
    b) Red blood cell
    c) Monocyte
    d) IgE
    e) Hepatocyte

11. Which one of the following statements is FALSE with regard to chronic urticaria?
    a) Defined as urticaria that persists for longer than 6 weeks
    b) Characterised by hives or wheals
    c) The mast cell is the primary agent in the pathogenesis of urticarial
    d) It is commonly due to urticarial vasculitis
    e) Non-sedating antihistamines are the mainstay of treatment

12. The following are all granulomatous conditions EXCEPT:
    a) Sarcoidosis
    b) Tuberculosis
    c) Pyogenic granuloma
    d) Histoplasmosis
    e) Schistosomiasis

13. Which two features are NOT parts of the nephrotic syndrome?
    a) Heavy proteinuria
    b) Microalbuminuria
    c) Oedema
    d) Hyperalbuminaemia
    e) Hypoalbuminaemia

14. Which two of the following statements are NOT true of non-Hodgkin lymphoma (NHL)?
    a) NHL is malignant proliferation of B cells
    b) NHL is curable and most cases are treatable
    c) The aetiological factors for NHL are largely unknown
    d) New cases of NHL are now becoming less frequent
    e) NHL does not have anaemia as a feature

15. Which of the following clinical features does NOT occur in thrombocytopenia?
    a) Purpura
    b) Menorrhagia
    c) Excess clotting
    d) Nose bleeds
    e) Gastrointestinal bleeding

Extended matching questions

Question 1
Choose the most appropriate answer from the list below:
a) CD4 cells
b) RNA retrovirus
c) DNA double-stranded helix
d) Seroconversion
e) CD3 cells
f) Malaise
g) Fever
h) Asymptomatic
i) Persistent generalised lymphadenopathy
j) ELISA testing
k) AIDS-related complex
l) Leishmaniasis
m) CMV
n) Lyme disease

1. A 40-year-old man, who migrated from Africa one year earlier, presents with dry, warty lesions of the skin as well as fevers, sweating, epistaxis and abdominal pain. He has known HIV-positive status. What is the most likely diagnosis?
2. What kind of virus is HIV and which cell receptor does it bind?
3. A 38-year-old man presents with symptoms of fever, malaise, myalgia, pharyngitis, a maculopapular rash and persistent oral *Candida*. He had unprotected sexual intercourse with a new partner 4 weeks earlier. What is the term used to describe his condition?

Question 2
Pick the correct responses from the following list:
a) Anti-Mi2
b) Anti-Jo1
c) Rh F
d) Anti-La (SSB)
e) Anti-RNP
f) Anti-Scl 70
g) AMA
h) ANTI-Ro (SSA)
i) SMA
j) Intrinsic factor Ab
k) Anti-endomysial Ab
l) C-ANCA
m) P-ANCA
n) Thyroid peroxidase Ab
o) Anti-double-stranded DNA

1. A 40-year-old Caucasian woman, who has a BMI in the obese range, presents with fatigue and pruritis. Clinical examination reveals hepatomegaly and blood tests show a raised alkaline phosphatase. What is the immune dysfunction in this patient?
2. A 51-year-old woman with known rheumatoid arthritis presents to her GP with new symptoms of dry mouth and dry eyes. Which two of the above are characteristic of this patient's presentation?
3. A 39-year-old woman presents with fatigue, weight loss, fever and malaise for some months. On examination she appears to have a malar flush across her face. Which one of the above is most specific for this condition?

Question 3
Choose the most appropriate response from the following list of vaccinations:
a) Measles
b) *Hemophilus influenzae* type B
c) Mumps
d) Influenza
e) Chickenpox
f) Meningococcal C
g) BCG
h) Rubella
i) Hib
j) Tetanus
k) Acellular pertussis
l) HPV
m) Inactivated polio
n) Diphtheria
o) Pneumococcal conjugate vaccine

1. Which six of the above options are given at two months after birth?
2. Which of the above is recommended to girls in the 12–18 age range?
3. Which three of the above options are recommended for all children at school-leaving age?

Answers

Single best answer questions

Q1 e.
The presence of blast cells on a blood film indicates leukaemia. In this patient this is acute leukaemia and is a medical emergency. She needs urgent same-day assessment.

Q2 c or d.
Any child with very frequent, difficult-to-treat or strange infections due to unusual organisms should be referred for a specialist opinion to exclude an immunodeficiency. Immunodeficiency syndromes can be classified according to the component of the immune system affected: T cells, B cells, phagocytic cells and complement.

Q3 e.
Selective IgA deficiency causes variable symptoms and most patients are only mildly affected. Other B-cell deficiencies include congenital X-linked hypogammaglobulinaemia and common variable immunodeficiency.

Q4 e.
In liver disease, IgM may be raised in primary biliary cirrhosis; alcohol may increase IgA levels; and autoimmune hepatitis causes rises in IgA and IgG. In sarcoidosis, IgA and IgG increase while IgM is usually normal.

Q5 b or d.
An occupational cause must be excluded in view of first onset of symptoms. Treatment is with emollients and steroids but the underlying cause must be identified. You should take a full occupational history: does she work with animals or wear latex gloves?

Q6 b.
There are four types of hypersensitivity reaction. Type I is immediate and includes anaphylaxis. Type II is antibody-dependent and includes autoimmune disorders such as Goodpasture syndrome and autoimmune haemolytic anaemia and are mediated by IgM or IgG. Type III is an immune complex hypersensitivity: it may be general (serum sickness) or may involve localised organs (e.g. the skin in systemic lupus erythematosus). Type IV is cell-mediated or delayed type hypersensitivity and is T-cell mediated.

Q7 d.
The history suggests C1 esterase inhibitor deficiency which causes hereditary angioedema. This is autosomal dominant. Patients present with angioedema but no urticaria. C4 is a useful screen: it is absent during acute attacks. A normal C4 during an attack excludes C1-esterase inhibitor deficiency. In this case the patient is not presenting acutely, so C1 esterase would be more useful. If urticaria was present, the diagnosis would not be C1-esterase inhibitor deficiency.

Q8 b.
IgA is the most common specific immunoglobulin deficiency (1 : 500–700). Although many with the condition are entirely asymptomatic, some patients may present with recurrent upper and lower respiratory tract infections. It is important to be aware that selective IgA deficiency is more prevalent in patients with autoimmune and collagen vascular diseases (rheumatoid arthritis, systemic lupus erythematosus, Sjögren syndrome, thyroiditis, coeliac disease). Treatment is with antibiotics for the underlying bacterial infection.

Q9 e.
The plasma concentration of serum amyloid A, CRP, ferritin and ceruloplasmin will increase in response to inflammation. Collectively, they are defined as 'positive' acute phase proteins; the examples given all act to inhibit or destroy the growth of microbes. Conversely, albumin is considered a 'negative' acute phase protein as plasma concentration of the protein will fall in response to inflammation.

Q10 c.
The term phagocyte originates from the Greek *phagein,* 'to devour' and *cyte* 'cell'. Other cells within this subgroup include neutrophils, macrophages and dendritic cells. These white blood cells are essential for fighting infection (as part of the innate immune system) and developing subsequent immunity (antigen presentation by dendritic cells).

Q11 d.
Urticaria is not strictly a disease but more a reaction pattern which represents cutaneous mast cell degradation, resulting in extravasation of plasma into the dermis. The primary subgroups of chronic urticaria are: physical urticaria; urticaria secondary to an underlying medical condition (it is rare for this condition to be the sole manifestation of a wider medical disease); and chronic idiopathic urticaria. Urticaria affects 15–20% of the population at some point in their lives, but the urticaria persists for more than 6 weeks (chronic urticaria) in only approximately 1% of the population. Antihistamines remain the mainstay of treatment.

Urticarial vasculitis is within the list of differential diagnosis of chronic uriticaria. It is a *forme fruste* of leukocytoclastic vasculitis (urticarial vasculitis clinically resembles urticaria but histologically show changes of leukocytoclastic vasculitis). Urticarial vasculitis may be associated with hypocomplementaemia and systemic symptoms.

Q12 c.
Pyogenic granuloma is one of the many known medical misnomers as it is neither pyogenic nor a granuloma. The condition is a benign, acquired vascular tumour of the skin and mucous membranes which presents as a rapidly growing vascular nodule or papule. The tumour

has a predilection for the head and neck and is often observed in infancy and childhood.

A granuloma is an organised collection of macrophages which form a 'tight ball' to wall off substances that are considered foreign but cannot be eliminated. Granulomas usually form in response to antigens that are resistant to 'first-responder' inflammatory cells such as neutrophils and eosinophils.

Q13 b, d.
Nephrotic syndrome is the presentation of renal disease which results from excessive protein loss. It is defined as the triad of heavy proteinuria (> 3 g in 24 hours), hypoalbuminaemia (< 25 g/L) and oedema. The reduced serum protein causes reduced plasma oncotic pressure which leads to oedema in patients.

Q14 d, e.
NHL can present as anaemia, recurrent infection or purpura, as well as the classic B symptoms of weight loss, night sweats and pyrexia.

The incidence of this condition is increasing though the reason for this is unknown.

Q15 c.
Thrombocytopenia is defined as less than 100×10^9/L platelets in the blood count. Patients have fewer platelets than is normal, and therefore are less able to clot effectively, leading to increased bleeding.

Extended matching questions
Question 1
Q1 i.
Leishmaniasis is a condition that is transmitted by sandflies. The condition can be visceral or cutaneous. The condition causes granulomata to form within the tissues with resulting sequelae. This clinical picture describes visceral leishmaniasis which can be HIV-associated. Incubation can be months to years.

Q2 b, a.
Human immunodeficiency virus is an RNA retrovirus that binds the CD4 cell receptor and causes cell destruction. As the rate of cell destruction outstrips cell replacement, the immune system becomes compromised and AIDS (acquired immune deficiency syndrome) develops.

Q3 d.
Acute seroconversion illness is the primary infection associated with HIV infection. This syndrome occurs around 2–6 weeks after virus exposure. The patient is diagnosed with AIDS if they present with an AIDS-defining illness. Patients can develop AIDS anywhere from 1 to 9 years after seroconversion.

Question 2

Q1 g.
This clinical picture is typical of patients with primary biliary cirrhosis. This condition develops as a result of an autoimmune response. A high percentage of patients have anti-mitochondrial antibodies; patients can however demonstrate anti-Ro, ANA as well as other autoantibodies classically associated with other syndromes. It is however the combination of clinical symptoms and signs as well as blood testing which makes the diagnosis.

Q2 d, h.
This patient has the classic combination of rheumatoid arthritis, xerostomia and keratoconjuntivitis sicca, known as Sjögren syndrome. This is a systemic autoimmune condition that attacks the exocrine function of the salivary glands and the tear ducts. The majority of patients affected are women and patients tend to be in their 40s to 50s.

Sjögren syndrome can develop as a primary condition or as part of another syndrome. It is associated with rheumatoid arthritis, systemic lupus erythematosus, scleroderma and primary biliary cirrhosis.

Q3 o.
The clinical features described in this case are typical of systemic lupus erythematosus. It is a non-organ-specific autoimmune condition that can have vasculitic, cutaneous or CNS features. Anti-dsDNA is the most specific autoantibody for systemic lupus erythematosus, though less specific antibodies such as anti-sm and anti-Ro can also be found.

Question 3

Q1 n, j, k, m, b, o.
The immunisation schedule for babies is as follows:

Birth	BCG to those at high risk
2 months	Combined vaccine (diphtheria, tetanus, acellular pertussis, inactivated polio, Hemophilus influenza type B and pneumococcal conjugate vaccine)
3 months	DTaP/IPV/Hib/meningococcal C
4 months	DTaP/IPV/Hib/Men C/pneumococcal conjugate vaccine

Q2 i.
The HPV vaccine is now offered to girls aged 12–13 and currently also targets girls from 13 to 18.

Q3 n, j, m.
This vaccine is offered in school, or at the time of school leaving.

9 Infectious Diseases

For each question below, what is the most likely answer?
Select one or more options from the answers supplied.

1. Which of the following infections is the cause of Lyme disease?
   a) *Treponema pallidum*
   b) *Borrelia burgdoferi*
   c) *Leptospira interrogans*
   d) *Treponema carateum*
   e) *Streptobacillus moniliformis*

2. Which of the following is a major criterion in rheumatic fever?
   a) Erythema marginatum
   b) Erythema migrans
   c) Fever
   d) Raised erythrocyte sedimentation rate or C-reactive protein
   e) ECG showing features of heart block, such as a prolonged PR interval

3. Considering treatment for symptomatic rabies, which statement is correct?
   a) Despite treatment rabies is usually fatal
   b) Doxycycline is the treatment of choice
   c) Erythromycin is the treatment of choice
   d) All patients should be given rabies immunoglobulin as soon as possible
   e) Intravenous teicoplanin

4. Which of the following is the most common cause of travellers' diarrhoea?
   a) *Campylobacter jejuni*
   b) *Shigella*

The Complete GPVTS Stage 2 Preparation Guide: Questions and Professional Dilemmas, First Edition. Edited by Saba Khan with Neel Sharma.
© 2012 John Wiley & Sons, Ltd. Published 2012 by John Wiley & Sons, Ltd.

c) *Salmonella*
d) *Giardia lamblia*
e) Enterotoxin-forming *Escherichia coli*

5. Which one of the following should result in exclusion of a child from school?
   a) A child with a rash from parvovirus B19 infection
   b) Chickenpox rash over a week, where the lesions have scabbed over
   c) Bacterial conjunctivitis
   d) Molluscum contagiosum
   e) Impetigo

6. Regarding threadworm infection, which statement is incorrect?
   a) Strict hygiene measures alone for 6 weeks can be used to clear up a threadworm infection
   b) Mebendazole is the preferred treatment option for children over 2 years of age
   c) Mebendazole can be bought over the counter
   d) All members of your household should be treated, even if only one person notices symptoms
   e) Should result in exclusion from school or nursery

7. Which of the following is NOT a major cause of iron deficiency anaemia?
   a) Malaria
   b) Hookworms
   c) Whipworms
   d) Roundworms
   e) Threadworms

8. Which TWO infections are of major concern if contracted in pregnancy?
   a) Malaria
   b) Group B streptococcus
   c) Gonorrhoea
   d) Toxoplasmosis
   e) *Clostridium difficile*

9. *Clostridium difficile* infection can be treated with which one of the following?
   a) Ciprofloxacin orally
   b) Vancomycin intravenously
   c) Cephalosporins
   d) Clindamycin
   e) Metronidazole orally

10. Which is the most common form of malarial infection?
    a) *Plasmodium ovale*

    b) *Plasmodium falciparum*

    c) *Plasmodium vivax*

    d) *Plasmodium knowlesi*

    e) *Plasmodium malariae*

11. Which is the single best answer regarding genital herpes infections?
    a) Genital herpes is a chronic, life-long infection
    b) In genital herpes infection, HSV-2 causes more than 90% of cases
    c) Rarely presents with a urethral discharge
    d) Is cured by used of antiviral medication, e.g. aciclovir
    e) Prevalence is estimated at 10% of the UK population

12. Which one of the following conditions is NOT a complication of varicella zoster infection?
    a) Erysipelas
    b) Encephalitis
    c) Myocarditis
    d) Hepatitis
    e) Splenomegaly

13. Which is the most common cause of hepatitis C infection?
    a) Sharing contaminated needles, spoons and filters to inject drugs
    b) Transmitted during unprotected sexual intercourse with an infected person
    c) Transfusion with infected blood or blood products, haemodialysis, or transplantation of organs from infected donors
    d) Needle-stick injury with HCV-contaminated blood, most commonly seen in healthcare workers
    e) From mother to infant at the time of childbirth

14. Which two of the following conditions do NOT have a vaccination for prevention of infection?
    a) Hepatitis B
    b) Hepatitis C
    c) Meningitis C
    d) Tuberculosis
    e) Leprosy

15. Which one of the following is NOT a major route of transmission for HIV?
    a) Contaminated needles
    b) Unprotected sex
    c) Breast milk
    d) Blood transfusions
    e) Perinatal transmission

Extended matching questions

Question 1
Pick one or more options from the following list to answer the questions.
a) Lungs
b) Eyes
c) Central nervous system
d) Genitourinary system
e) Gastrointestinal system
f) Lymphatic system
g) Red
h) Blue
i) Green
j) Rifampicin
k) Streptomycin
l) Ethambutol
m) Isoniazid
n) Hydrazine

1. A patient is admitted to hospital with possible TB infection. He is isolated and investigations are ordered. One of the lab tests involves Ziehl–Neelson staining of the patient's sputum. What colour do the acid-fast bacilli stain with this test?
2. A 32-year-old man presents with known TB, he has not however taken any treatment at all as he felt he would recover on his own. He is now feeling considerably worse and has developed several new symptoms. Which three systems are most likely to be affected by extrapulmonary TB?
3. A 32-year-old patient is admitted to hospital and confirmed to have TB. Which two agents could be used as first-line therapy for this disease?

Question 2
Choose one or more options from the following list to answer the questions below:
a) Influenza virus A
b) Influenza virus B
c) Influenza virus C
d) Reddened skin, eyes and mouth
e) Pale skin
f) Fever
g) Rigors
h) Diarrhoea
i) Chronic asthma patients
j) Diabetes patients
k) Adolescents
l) Patients undergoing stress
m) Children

1. Influenza virus affects humans, birds and mammals. Which species of virus is the most virulent in humans?
2. A 26-year-old woman presents with influenza symptoms to her GP. Which three symptoms is she most likely to have?
3. Which three groups of patients are classed as being at high risk from influenza infection and therefore are eligible for the influenza vaccine?

Question 3

Choose one or more options from the following list in answer to the questions below.

a) Unknown cause
b) Infection
c) Neoplastic disease
d) Connective tissue disease
e) Daily spikes of fever
f) Saddleback fever
g) Spikes of fever that occur twice in the day
h) Continuous fever with some variation
i) Occupation
j) Hobbies
k) Travel
l) People contacts
m) Pets
n) Sexual contact

1. From the list above, choose the two most likely findings in patients with fever of unknown origin (PUO).
2. A 47-year-old man has been admitted to hospital with PUO. He has had various investigations and has been diagnosed with an abscess. What pattern of fever might you expect him to have displayed?
3. A patient presents with very high fevers, severe headache focused retro-orbitally, significant redness to the face, severe myalgia and a diffuse maculopapular rash.
   Which question would be most pertinent to the patient history?

Answers

Single best answer questions
Q1 b.
The cause of Lyme disease is *Borrelia burgdoferi*. *Treponema pallidum* causes syphilis, while *Treponema carateum* causes pinta, a skin condition found in Mexico, Central and South America. It is morphologically and serologically indistinguishable from the organism that causes syphilis. *Leptospira interrogans* is the organism responsible for Weil disease. *Streptobacillus moniliformis* is a cause of rat bite fever.

Q2 a.
Erythema marginatum is the presence of pink rings on the trunk and inner surfaces of the limbs, which come and go for several months. It is found primarily on extensor surfaces occurs in less than 5% of patients with rheumatic fever, but is considered a major Jones criterion when it does occur. The four other major criteria are carditis, polyarthritis, Sydenham chorea and subcutaneous nodules.

Erythema migrans is found in Lyme disease, while answers c, d and e are minor criteria for rheumatic fever.

Q3 a.
Rabies is a classic 'zoonosis', it is an illness that is passed directly from animal to animal and from animal to human. The virus that causes rabies is a Lyssavirus. Once visible symptoms have developed, the mortality rate is almost 100%. Very few people are known to have survived a rabies infection.

Treatment is both by giving specific immunoglobulin (passive immunisation) and by administration of a normal vaccination (active immunisation). Patients who have previously received pre-exposure vaccination do not receive the immunoglobulin, only the post-exposure vaccinations on day 0 and 3.

Q4 a.
Travellers' diarrhoea is usually contracted by the ingestion of contaminated food or water. Most cases of travellers' diarrhoea are caused by bacteria. The most important bacterium is enterotoxigenic *E. coli* which is estimated to account for up to 70% of all cases.

Other bacterial species implicated in travellers' diarrhoea include *Campylobacter jejuni, Shigella* and *Salmonella*. Parasitic infections are an uncommon cause with the exception of *Giardia lamblia* and *Cryptosporidium*.

Q5 e.
Active impetigo would require a child to be excluded from school. Patients are infectious when developing the rash in parvovirus, and for 1 week in

chickenpox once the rash appears. Bacterial conjunctivitis is not highly contagious, and molluscum infection is a chronic childhood condition which requires no treatment.

Q6 e.

Threadworms (*Enterobius vermicularis*) are small worm parasites that infect the intestines of humans. Threadworms do not always cause symptoms, although some patients can experience itching around the anus and vagina. The itchiness is particularly noticeable at night and can disturb sleep.

The Health Protection Agency (HPA) advises that children should still go to school if they have a threadworm infection. Schools and nurseries should follow good hygiene practices to limit the spread of infection.

Q7 e.

Worldwide, the most important cause of iron deficiency anaemia is parasitic infection caused by hookworms, whipworms and roundworms, where intestinal bleeding caused by the worms can lead to undetected blood loss in the stool. This is especially important in growing children. Chronic blood loss caused by hookworms and malaria infections contributes to anaemia during pregnancy in most developing countries. Threadworms cause loss of appetite and weight loss, but not iron deficient anaemia.

Q8 a, d.

Malarial infection during pregnancy is a major public health problem in tropical and subtropical regions of the world. In these areas maternal death may result either directly from severe malaria or indirectly from malaria-related severe anaemia. In addition, malaria infection of the mother may result in a range of adverse pregnancy outcomes, including spontaneous abortion, neonatal death and low birth weight (LBW).

Toxoplasmosis infection may lead to miscarriage, stillbirth, or survival with growth problems, blindness, water on the brain (hydrocephalus), brain damage, epilepsy or deafness.

Q9 e.

Antibiotic-associated colitis is an infection of the colon caused by *C. difficile* that occurs primarily among individuals who have been using antibiotics. The use of antibiotics causes eradication of the normal gut flora with proliferation of *C. difficile* leading to pseudo-membranous colitis.

Oral metronidazole is the first-line treatment. Intravenous vancomycin has no effect on *C. difficile* colitis since the antibiotic is not excreted appreciably into the colon. However, oral vancomycin can be used in more severe infections as it is not absorbed from the gut and hence is effective in treating the *Clostridium* infection.

Q10 b.

Plasmodium falciparum is the most common cause of infection, and results in 80% of all malaria cases, and is also responsible for about 90% of the deaths from malarial infection.

There are four other types of malaria parasite: *Plasmodium vivax*, *Plasmodium ovale* and *Plasmodium malariae* cause more benign types of malaria; *Plasmodium knowlesi* is an emerging species that causes malaria in monkeys, but rarely can also infect humans.

Q11 a.

Genital herpes is caused by the herpes simplex virus (HSV). There are two types: HSV-1 and HSV-2. Most genital herpes infections were thought to be caused by HSV-2; however, cases due to HSV-1 are now approximately equal, with a prevalence of genital herpes estimated at 1 in 4 in the UK.

In most cases, genital herpes is a chronic (long-term) condition. Many people with HSV have frequently recurring genital herpes, recurring an average of four to five times in the first two years after being infected. However, the incidence of genital herpes decreases over time, and the condition becomes less severe with each subsequent occurrence. Symptoms include painful red blisters, urethral discharge and dysuria, with flares treated with antiviral medications which include aciclovir.

Q12 e.

Chickenpox (varicella zoster) is usually an infection of childhood that runs a self-limiting course. However, rarely and in particular in those who are immunocompromised, more serious complications can occur.

Other serious sequelae include varicella pneumonia and haemorrhagic chickenpox.

Q13 a.

Sharing of contaminated needles among injecting drug users is the most common mode of transmission.

Transfusion with infected blood or blood products, haemodialysis, or transplantation of organs from infected donors was once a common mode of transmission but is now rare following the implementation in 1992 of HCV blood testing for all donor blood and blood products.

The risk of developing HCV infection after a needle-stick injury is about 5–10%. There is a small (1 in 20) risk that a mother who is infected with the hepatitis C virus will pass the infection on to her baby.

Q14 b, e.

Though hepatitis A and B have vaccinations, none are available for hepatitis C or leprosy.

BCG immunisation protects against tuberculosis; however, it is no longer routinely administered in the UK since 2005, instead focusing on high-risk groups.

There is a Hib vaccine, a meningitis C vaccine, and most recently a vaccine to protect against pneumoccoccal meningitis as part of the routine immunisation programme in the UK. However, there is still no vaccine to protect against all forms of meningitis and associated diseases, including the most common in the UK: meningococcal group B and streptococcal group B.

Q15 d.
While all answers are a potential route of HIV transmission, blood product screening has largely eliminated transmission of HIV through this method; however, in the developing world systems are not always as effective. In more poverty-stricken regions of the world, perinatal and breast milk transmission play a much larger role.

Extended matching questions
Question 1
Q1 g.
On Ziehl–Neelson staining the acid-fast bacilli appear red against a blue background. Fluorescent microscopy can also be used to identify the bacterium.

Q2 c, d, f.
Patients can develop meningitis, scrofula of the neck from lymph infection and significant damage to the urogenital tract dependent on where the focus of infection lies. Patients can also develop Pott disease, which is caused by abscess formation in the spine.

Q3 j, m.
Rifampicin and isoniazid are first-line agents in TB. If patients do not take treatment as directed they can develop multidrug-resistant TB which then requires further treatment and management by specialist services.

Question 2
Q1 a.
Influenza virus A is the most virulent strain and causes the most severe disease. It is naturally found in aquatic birds but can cause infection in humans with resulting pandemics.

Q2 d, f, g.
Patients may also experience body aches, cough, nasal congestion and headache. Children with influenza are more likely to experience abdominal pain and diarrhoea. Some may even have vomiting.

Q3 i, j, m.

The elderly and patients who are immunocompromised are also in the high-risk group.

Question 3

Q1 a, b.

Pharmacotherapy and abscess formation may also result in PUO; however, the majority are as a result of infection or the cause remains unknown.

Q2 e.

Daily spikes of fever are also seen in TB. Saddleback fever occurs where patients have more tropical infection such as dengue fever or legionnaires' disease. This results in fever for a few days which resolves for a few days and then returns again.

Spiking fever twice a day is seen in leishmaniasis, and continuous fever with fluctuations is seen in malaria.

These causes are not exhaustive but demonstrate the diagnostic capacity for symptom patterns.

Q3 k.

This patient demonstrates the classic presentation for dengue fever; the fever is also typically saddleback. Patients may also exhibit more serious features such as haemorrhage from the nose, gums or gastrointestinal tract or with menorrhagia. Patients may have been to countries in Asia or South America.

10 Musculoskeletal Disorders

For each question below, what is the most likely answer?
Select ONE option only from the answers supplied.

1. Which one of the following is NOT commonly found in limited systemic sclerosis?
   a) Telangiectasia
   b) Sclerodactyly
   c) Calcinosis
   d) Oesophageal dysfunction
   e) Exophthalmos

2. A patient presents to your surgery after a fall with pain in their right shoulder. After a full examination, you find that they have restricted abduction of the arm between 0 and 90 degrees. Which tendon is most likely to be affected?
   a) Infraspinatus tendon
   b) Subscapularis tendon
   c) Supraspinatus tendon
   d) Teres minor tendon
   e) Biceps tendon

3. A 73-year-old woman presents to your surgery complaining of gradually worsening pain and stiffness in her neck, shoulders and both hips. The pain is worse in the mornings and she feels constantly tired. On examination, there is no associated muscle weakness but you discover she has a right-sided carpal tunnel syndrome. Investigations reveal a mildly elevated CRP and ESR with a negative rheumatoid factor. What is the most likely diagnosis?
   a) Polymyalgia rheumatica
   b) Rheumatoid arthritis
   c) Osteoarthritis

The Complete GPVTS Stage 2 Preparation Guide: Questions and Professional Dilemmas, First Edition. Edited by Saba Khan with Neel Sharma.
© 2012 John Wiley & Sons, Ltd. Published 2012 by John Wiley & Sons, Ltd.

d) Pseudogout

e) Polymyositis

4. A 77-year-old patient presents in the Emergency Department after a fall; you suspect a Colles fracture and send the patient for an X-ray. Which one of the following statements is FALSE with regard to this particular fracture type?

a) The fracture involves the distal radius

b) There is volar (anterior) displacement of the distal fragment

c) The patient usually gives a history of falling onto an outstretched hand

d) It can be associated with a fracture of the ulnar styloid

e) Radial shortening is a recognised radiographic finding

5. A 57-year-old woman with known rheumatoid arthritis (RA) presents to your clinic with shortness of breath. The following are recognised pulmonary complications of rheumatoid arthritis EXCEPT:

a) Bronchiectasis

b) Pleural effusion

c) Obliterative bronchiolitis

d) Pulmonary fibrosis

e) Pneumothorax

6. A 35-year-old patient presents to the Emergency Department complaining of a constant pain in his right calf. He describes a sudden onset of pain while playing tennis, accompanied by an audible 'pop'. On examination, he is maximally tender in the right calf with radiation to the ankle; there is associated swelling and bruising of the calf. On further questioning, you find he has just returned from a 2-week holiday in Australia. What is the most likely cause for the patient's pain?

a) Gastrocnemius muscle injury

b) Deep vein thrombosis

c) Acute arterial occlusion

d) Achilles tendon rupture

e) Popliteal artery entrapment syndrome

7. A 65-year-old woman presents to your clinic with bilateral knee pain. The pain originally began a year ago with a now notable worsening of symptoms. She awakes with stiffness in the knees and a gradual worsening of the pain as the day progresses. On examination, you notice she has a mild deformity and tenderness of a number of the distal interphalangeal (DIP) joints in both hands. On asking her to walk, you discover crepitus of the left knee. The likely diagnosis is?

a) Rheumatoid arthritis

b) Haemochromatosis

c) Psoriatic arthropathy

d) Osteoarthritis

e) Ankylosing spondylitis

8. A 27-year-old man comes to your clinic with a painful second toe. You check his patient records and find he has presented to the surgery before with dysuria and was given antibiotics for a presumed 'urinary tract infection'. He has also seen an ophthalmologist recently with redness of the right eye. On further questioning, he remembers having a bout of bloody diarrhoea before the onset of his symptoms. He has no known chronic illness and no other symptoms than those described. On examination of his feet, you find the toe to be diffusely swollen, red, hot and tender to touch. Which one of the following is the most likely diagnosis?
a) Enteropathic arthritis
b) Ankylosing spondylitis
c) Reactive arthritis
d) Gonococcal arthritis
e) Osteomyelitis

9. A 70-year-old man has had five episodes of right knee pain and swelling. Most of the episodes resolve within a few days, with the longest attack lasting a maximum of 7 days. He is completely asymptomatic between attacks, with ibuprofen 400 mg (taken at regular intervals) usually relieving his symptoms. His most recent episode was 2 months ago. On examination, his knee is not swollen or tender but there is marked crepitus on knee extension, as well as a moderate suprapatellar joint effusion. Which one of the following tests would confirm the diagnosis?
a) Arthrocentesis of the knee with analysis of the fluid
b) Knee radiograph
c) Ultrasound of the knee
d) MRI of the knee
e) Measurement of serum uric acid

10. A 65-year-old man has come to your surgery to discuss the result of his recently taken ankle radiographs. He originally presented 2 weeks ago with bilateral ankle pain and was seen by your colleague. You look through his notes and discover the radiology report which comments on a periosteal reaction and suggests a diagnosis of hypertrophic osteoarthropathy. Which of the following is the next most appropriate step for the management of this patient?
a) Reassure the patient he has a degenerative condition and prescribe some analgesia for his pain
b) Order a radionuclide study of both legs
c) Order a chest radiograph
d) Order an MRI and refer him for an orthopaedic opinion
e) Order thyroid function tests

11. A 35-year-old patient presents with frank haemoptysis. Within the last two months, he has had recurrent episodes of epistaxis and sinusitis. On examination, you find the nasal septum has been destroyed

causing a 'saddle-nose' deformity; there is also a proptosis of the left eye. Laboratory studies reveal Hb 12.1 g/dL and WBC 9 × 10⁹/L. Urinalysis is performed and tests positive for protein. Which of the following tests will help achieve the diagnosis?
a) Measurement of antiglomerular basement membrane antibody
b) Measurement of antineutrophil cytoplasmic antibody
c) Measurement of rheumatoid factor
d) Chest X-ray
e) Toxicology screen

12. The following is NOT a recognised side effect of corticosteroid therapy (prednisolone):
a) Proximal myopathy
b) Reduced appetite
c) Peptic ulceration
d) Avascular osteonecrosis
e) Osteoporosis

13. The following are all recognised risk factors for osteoporosis EXCEPT:
a) Smoking
b) Low levels of physical activity
c) Family history
d) Early menarche
e) Hyperparathyroidism

14. A 65-year-old woman presents with a constant back pain. You send her for some preliminary blood tests and find she has a raised ESR (70 mm/hr) and calcium (3.1 mmol/L), a normochromic normocytic anaemia (10.2 g/dL) and normal alkaline phosphatase (ALP) levels. What is the most likely diagnosis?
a) Paget disease
b) Myeloma
c) Osteoporosis
d) Osteomalacia
e) Pott's disease

15. Which of the following is NOT true with regard to Jaccoud arthropathy?
a) Is associated with marginal erosions
b) Can involve the wrists and hands
c) Causes ulnar deviation
d) Is observed in patients with systemic lupus erythematosus
e) Is associated with subluxation of the metacarpophalangeal (MCP) joints

Extended matching questions

Question 1

For each of the following scenarios select the SINGLE best answer from the list below:

a) Haemochromatosis
b) Rheumatoid arthritis
c) Osteoarthritis
d) Calcium pyrophosphate dehydrate (CPPD) arthropathy
e) Gout
f) Psoriatic arthritis
g) Polymyositis
h) Reactive arthritis
i) Gonococcal septicaemia
j) Enteropathic arthritis
k) Ankylosing spondylitis
l) Systemic lupus erythematosus
m) Dermatomyositis

1. A 45-year-old man presents to your surgery having just moved into the local area. He has a known chronic condition which he refers to as a 'problem with my bones'. His main concerns are a back pain which is worse at night with marked morning stiffness and a pain and swelling of his left heel. On examination, he is kyphotic with a clear hyperextension of the neck. Spinal movement is restricted in all directions. Auscultation reveals a high-pitched early diastolic murmur, best heard in expiration and with the patient sitting forward. Of the above, which is the most likely diagnosis?
2. A 75-year-old patient has come to your clinic for a follow-up appointment. On her last visit she had complained of right knee pain with an associated joint effusion. You had sent her for a radiograph of her knees (which demonstrated chondrocalcinosis) and had aspirated her effusion. Polarised light microscopy analysis of the aspirate reveals weakly positively birefringent crystals. What is the most likely diagnosis?
3. A 35-year-old patient presents with malaise, myalgia and a migratory asymmetric polyarthropathy with an upper extremity predominance. On examination, you note she has a tenosynovitis affecting the dorsum of the wrist and a painless, nonpruritic rash consisting of pustules, small papules and vesicles. Multiple joints are found to be red, hot and swollen. What is the likely diagnosis?

Question 2

For each of the following scenarios select the SINGLE best answer from the list below:

a) Perthes disease
b) Osgood–Schlatter disease
c) Slipped upper femoral epiphysis (SUFE)
d) Scaphoid fracture
e) Posterior dislocation of the shoulder
f) Metacarpal fracture
g) Hook of hamate fracture
h) Developmental dysplasia of the hip (DDH)
i) Osteochondritis dissecans
j) Anterior dislocation of the shoulder
k) Acromioclavicular dislocation
l) Greenstick fracture
m) Fracture of neck of femur

1. A known epileptic presents in the Emergency Department after a
   tonic–clonic seizure. He complains of a right shoulder pain; he is
   holding his arm in adduction and internal rotation. What is the most
   likely diagnosis?
2. An 8-year-old boy is brought to your surgery complaining of pain in
   the right hip with an associated limp. The mother tells you the
   symptoms have been gradually worsening over the last few weeks. On
   examination, there is slight restriction of movement on internal
   rotation. Which option from the above list is the most likely diagnosis?
3. A 19-year-old male presents to your surgery with a painful hand after
   punching a wall. He refuses an examination because of pain. You send
   him for an X-ray of the hand and wrist on which a fracture is identified.
   From the list above, select the most likely fracture type identified in this
   mode of injury.

Question 3
For each of the following scenarios select the SINGLE best answer from
the list below:
a) Anterior cruciate ligament (ACL) tear
b) Posterior cruciate ligament (PCL) tear
c) Meniscal tear
d) Medial collateral ligament (MCL) injury
e) Lateral collateral ligament (LCL) injury
f) Iliotibial tract syndrome
g) Prepatellar bursitis
h) Baker's cyst
i) Patella dislocation
j) Osteoarthritis
k) Quadriceps tendon rupture
l) Supraspinatus tendinitis
m) Olecranon bursitis

1. A 40-year-old plumber attends your surgery with right knee pain and swelling. On examination, there is tenderness of the patella to palpation, with a fluctuant swelling over the lower pole of the patella and restricted knee flexion secondary to pain. The joint is normal. What is the most likely diagnosis?

2. A 21-year-old professional basketball player presents to you with a painful left knee. The pain initially occurred after he twisted his knee while playing in a qualifying match. Since then, the knee intermittently locks and occasionally feels like it is about to give way. On examination, there is joint line tenderness. What is the most likely diagnosis?

3. A 28-year-old long-jumper presents with left knee pain. The injury occurred two hours prior to his attendance and he recalls hearing a loud pop after completing his jump, soon after which he noticed a knee swelling. He has been in constant pain since. On examination, the 'anterior draw test' demonstrates an anterior translation of the tibia in relation to the femur of 1 cm, with a 6 mm degree of side-to-side displacement discerned using the Lachman test. What is the most likely diagnosis?

Answers

Single best answer questions

Q1 e.

The CREST syndrome (limited systemic sclerosis) comprises calcinosis (pathological calcification of the soft tissues), Raynaud phenomenon, (o)esophageal dysmotility, sclerodactyly (thickening of the skin of the digits of the hands and feet) and telangiectasia. Skin involvement is limited to the face, hands and feet. It is associated with anti-centromere antibodies (70–80%) and pulmonary hypertension.

Q2 c.

Collectively, the infraspinatus, subscapularis, supraspinatus and teres minor muscles and their tendons make up the rotator cuff and bring stability to the shoulder joint. It is often the tendons and not the muscles which are torn after traumatic injury. Pain in the 0–90 degree range of movement is due to supraspinatus tendon injury. Pain on internal rotation is due to subscapularis involvement, whereas pain on external rotation locates the injury to the infraspinatous +/− teres minor.

Q3 a.

Polymyalgia rheumatica is characterised by symmetric pain of the shoulder and hip girdles without associated weakness. The patient will often complain of prolonged morning stiffness, malaise and weight loss. The disease is common in those over 70 years and rare in those younger than 60 years. Carpal tunnel syndrome is coexistent in 10% of patients. CRP and ESR are usually raised, with steroids being the mainstay of treatment.

Q4 b.

Colles fractures usually occur in patients > 50 years of age who fall onto an outstretched hand resulting in a fracture of the distal radius with dorsal displacement of the distal fracture fragment. The recognised components of the fracture include: dorsal angulation and displacement of the distal fragment; radial deviation of the hand; comminution at the fracture site; radial shortening and loss of ulnar inclination. An associated fracture of the ulnar styloid is well recognised.

Q5 e.

Up to 10% of patients with rheumatoid arthritis may show radiographic signs of bronchiectasis and are more likely to be heterozygous for the CTFR mutation seen in cystic fibrosis. Clinically significant interstitial lung disease is thought to occur in 5–10% of patients with RA. Pneumothorax is not a recognised association.

Q6 a.

The given history of a sudden onset of pain within the calf with an accompanying audible 'pop' is characteristic of an injury to the medial head of the gastrocnemius muscle. An Achilles tendon rupture will result in the patient being unable to plantarflex the foot and a more distal defect is usually palpable. A Thompson test can be used to differentiate the two injuries. The test is performed with the patient prone and the knee held in flexion, after which the gastrocnemius muscle is squeezed. A negative sign results in normal plantarflexion of the foot and ankle. If the flexion is not appreciated, the test is positive and due to a disrupted Achilles tendon.

The given history and examination findings render the remaining options less likely. The recent history of travel is coincidental in this case.

Q7 d.

The most important discriminator in this scenario is the nature of pain. Mechanical pain, as in this case, usually has a short duration of morning stiffness with worsening of pain on use. Inflammatory pain (psoriasis, rheumatoid arthritis) usually has a longer duration of morning stiffness with the pain improving with activity. The DIP deformity identified is secondary to Heberden's nodes; the lack of any associated concomitant inflammatory findings makes psoriatic arthropathy less likely.

Q8 c.

Urethritis, arthritis and conjunctivitis are the classic triad associated with Reiter syndrome (now referred to as reactive arthritis). A sterile arthritis, which typically affects the lower limbs, occurring approximately 1–4 weeks after an initial episode of urethritis or dysentery is the typical natural history of the disease. Other clinical manifestations include iritis, keratoderma blenorrhagica, circinate balanitis, mouth ulcers and enthesitis. There is a known association with HLA-B27 (65–96% patient positivity); because of this and clinical overlap with ankylosing spondylitis and psoriatic arthritis, reactive arthritis is classified as a type of seronegative spondyloarthropathy.

Q9 a.

The history and examination findings suggest recurrent attacks of gout or pseudogout. The diagnosis is best attained by analysing crystals from the joint fluid aspirate. A high yield of crystals within the fluid can usually be expected, even in patients who are asymptomatic at the time of aspiration. Serum uric acid can be raised in people who do not have gout, with the converse also holding true. Underlying bony abnormalities can take years to manifest on a radiograph. Similarly, an ultrasound of the knee and MRI are unlikely to demonstrate any definitive diagnostic features of gout or pseudogout.

Q10 c.

Hypertrophic osteoarthropathy (HOA) is a clinical syndrome of clubbing of the fingers and toes, enlargement of the extremities and painful swollen joints. It is characterised by symmetric periostitis involving the radius and fibula and, to a lesser extent, the femur, humerus, metacarpals and metatarsals. The syndrome can be primary or secondary. Secondary causes of HOA can be subdivided into pleural, cardiac, pulmonary and abdominal:

- Pleural: fibrous tumour of the pleura and mesothelioma
- Cyanotic heart disease with a right-to-left shunt
- Pulmonary: lung cancer, pulmonary tuberculosis, abscess, blastomycosis, bronchiectasis, emphysema and *Pneumocystis carinii* pneumonia (PCP) infection in patients with AIDS, Hodgkin disease, metastases, or cystic fibrosis
- Abdominal causes include liver cirrhosis, ulcerative colitis, Crohn disease, gastrointestinal tract neoplasms (gastric and pancreatic), lymphoma of the bowel, Whipple disease and biliary atresia

Chest radiograph is therefore the next most appropriate management step, primarily to ascertain whether a primary lung carcinoma is present.

Q11 b.

The constellation of presenting symptoms and signs best supports a diagnosis of Wegener granulomatosis. The disease is characterised by a necrotising granulomatous inflammation and vasculitis of the small and medium-sized vessels. cANCA (antineutrophil cytoplasmic antibody) with a raised PR3 is found in the majority of patients. Upper airways disease is common, with ulcers, epistaxis, nasal septal destruction and sinusitis all recognised. Pulmonary involvement may manifest as a cough, pleuritis or haemoptysis. While a chest radiograph may demonstrate infiltrates, nodules, cavitations or consolidation from haemorrhage, it will not help specifically differentiate from other causes of such radiograph findings. Renal disease causes a rapidly progressive glomerulonephritis with crescent formation, proteinuria or haematuria. Ocular involvement is well documented with proptosis (due to retrobublar granulomas) occurring in 50% of patients.

Antiglomerular basement membrane antibodies are present in patients with Goodpasture syndrome. These patients will not have any sinus involvement. A toxicology screen should be ordered if cocaine abuse is suspected; however, the clinical findings in this particular scenario are inconsistent with this diagnosis.

Q12 b.

Corticosteroids will cause an *increased* appetite with weight gain.

Q13 d.

A reduced duration of exposure to oestrogens will increase the risk of developing osteoporosis. As such, an early menopause and a *late* menarche, as opposed to the converse, are recognised risk factors for this condition. Other risk factors include slender body habitus, alcohol consumption, steroids, amenorrhoea, vertebral deformity, low dietary calcium intake and malabsorbtion.

Coexistent medical conditions associated with a decrease in bone mass include: Cushing syndrome, thyrotoxicosis, myeloma, primary biliary cirrhosis, rheumatoid arthritis and mastocytosis.

Q14 b.

Myeloma is a malignant clonal proliferation of B-lymphocyte-derived plasma cells with a subsequent over-abundance of monoclonal paraprotein. Osteolytic bone lesions or vertebral collapse can be the cause of unexplained back pain and result in hypercalcaemia in approximately 40% of such patients. Anaemia is usually a consequence of marrow infiltration.

In Paget disease of the bone, the Ca^{2+} is normal, while the ALP is markedly raised; the serum Ca^{2+} and ALP are normal in osteoporosis; and in osteomalacia serum Ca^{2+} is usually reduced and ALP is raised.

Q15 a.

Jaccoud arthropathy (JA) is a *non-erosive*, deforming arthropathy of the metacarpophalangeal (MCP) and proximal interphalangeal (PIP) joints and the wrist. It was first described as a rare complication of recurrent rheumatic fever and is now more commonly associated with systemic lupus erythematosus (SLE). Hand deformities typically present with ulnar deviation and subluxation of the MCP, similar to that observed in rheumatoid arthritis. In JA, however, ligament laxity and muscle imbalance rather than the loss of bone and joint instability secondary to synovitis determine the clinical picture.

Extended matching questions
Question 1
Q1 k.

Ankylosing spondylitis (AS) is a chronic inflammatory condition of the spine and sacroiliac joints. Kyphosis and neck hypertension (described as a 'question mark posture'), as well as spino-cranial ankylosis are all recognised patterns of progression. Other features include enthestis, anterior uveitis, aortitis and aortic regurgitation, apical fibrosis and amyloidosis. AS is recognised as a seronegative spondyloarthropathy with > 95% of patients testing positive for HLA B27.

Q2 d.

CPPD (formerly known as pseudogout) can be an *acute* process, similar to gout, presenting as a monarthritis. The acute variant is usually spontaneous and self-limiting. Alternatively, the condition can be a more destructive *chronic* process similar to osteoarthritis. CPPD is associated with chondrocalcinosis and conditions such as hyperparathyroidism, haemochromatosis and hypothyroidism. Polarised light microscopy analysis of the aspirate revealing weakly positively birefringent crystals is diagnostic.

Q3 i.

The triad of migratory polyarthritis, tenosynovitis and dermatitis is well recognised in the bacteraemic variant of disseminated gonococcal infection. Gonococcal arthritis is caused by infection with the Gram-negative diplococcus *Neisseria gonorrhoeae*. In the United States, it is the most common form of septic arthritis; however, the condition is relatively rare in Western Europe. Joint involvement can be a result of the *bacteremic* form of the disease (as described in the scenario), or a *septic arthritis* form where patients may experience pain, redness and swelling in usually one or sometimes multiple joints, most commonly the knees, wrists, ankles and elbows.

Question 2

Q1 e.

Posterior dislocation of the shoulder is rare (< 2% of all shoulder dislocations). This type of injury is seen in patients post-seizure and after electric shocks. Patients usually present with their arm adducted and internally rotated with attempts at abduction and external rotation causing pain.

Q2 a.

Perthes disease is a disorder of the upper femoral epiphysis in which the growing epiphysis becomes ischaemic and infracted. The condition usually presents at age 7–8, although it may occur at any age from 3 years up to 11 or 12. Boys are affected more commonly than girls and about 15% of cases are bilateral. The radiograph changes are characteristic. SUFE usually presents in obese males of an older age group (10–17 years old).

Q3 f.

Fractures of the fourth/fifth metacarpal are referred to as 'brawler's fractures'.

Question 3

Q1 g.

The prepatellar bursa has a thin synovial lining and is superficially located between the skin and the patella. Prepatellar bursitis, also known as 'housemaid's knee', is due to inflammation of the prepatellar bursa. Aseptic prepatellar bursitis is associated with certain professions which require repetitive kneeling such as carpet fitters, plumbers, housemaids and coal miners.

Q2 c.

Meniscal injuries are the most frequent sporting injury to the knee joint. Injuries to the healthy meniscus are usually produced by compressive forces coupled with rotation of the flexed knee as it starts to move into extension. Locking is a common symptom. If the fragment becomes lodged momentarily in the knee joint, the patient may experience the sensation of the knee giving way. Joint line tenderness indicates injury in 77–86% of patients with meniscus tears.

Q3 a.

ACL injury may occur as a non-contact injury, where an audible 'pop' is often heard after changing direction, cutting, or landing from a jump. In a contact and high-energy setting, the injury is associated with other ligamentous injury, such as the MCL and medial meniscus.

The Lachman test is performed with the knee held in 20–30° of flexion. The femur is stabilised with the non-dominant hand, and an anteriorly directed force is applied to the calf. The amount of displacement (in mm) and the quality of endpoint are assessed. Asymmetry in side-to-side laxity (> 3 mm is considered abnormal) or a soft endpoint is indicative of an ACL tear.

The anterior draw test is performed with the knee flexed to 90°. The examiner usually sits on the patient's foot and holds the patient's calf with both hands. An anterior force is applied, and tibial excursion is compared to the unaffected knee. Excessive glide anteriorly (> 5 mm) implies ACL damage; excessive glide posteriorly implies PCL damage.

11 Neurology

For each question below, what is the most likely answer?
Select ONE option only from the answers supplied.

1. Which of those listed below is NOT a symptom of an upper motor neurone lesion?
   a) Spasticity
   b) Hyperreflexia
   c) Positive Babinski sign
   d) Negative Babinski sign
   e) Hoffman reflex

2. A middle cerebral artery occlusion would NOT cause which ONE of the following?
   a) Ipsilateral homonymous hemianopia
   b) Contralateral hemiparesis
   c) Dysphasia in dominant hemisphere lesions
   d) Visio-spatial disturbance
   e) Hemisensory loss

3. Which of the following is a serotonin antagonist?
   a) Sumatriptan
   b) Lithium
   c) Fluoxetine
   d) Buspirone
   e) Pizotifen

4. Which one of the following statements is INCORRECT in relation to movements testing for peripheral nerve damage?
   a) For nerve root C3, 4 – (trapezius), ask patient to shrug shoulders
   b) For nerve root C6, 7, 8 – (triceps), ask patient to extend the elbow against resistance

The Complete GPVTS Stage 2 Preparation Guide: Questions and Professional Dilemmas, First Edition. Edited by Saba Khan with Neel Sharma.
© 2012 John Wiley & Sons, Ltd. Published 2012 by John Wiley & Sons, Ltd.

c) For nerve root L2, 3, 4 – (quadriceps), ask patient to extend the knee against resistance

d) For nerve root L2, 3, 4 – (quadriceps), ask patient to flex the knee against resistance

e) For nerve root C6, 7, 8 – (latissimus dorsi), ask patient to adduct arm

5. Which of the following neurotransmitter receptors has as yet not been pharmacologically manipulated?
   a) Serotonin
   b) Adrenaline and noradrenaline
   c) Acetylcholine
   d) Dopamine
   e) Purines

6. Which ONE of the following symptoms is NOT a feature of an acute stroke?
   a) Contralateral flaccid hemiplegia
   b) Hemisensory loss
   c) Visio-spatial neglect
   d) Homonymous hemianopia
   e) Spasticity

7. Which of the following is NOT a part of the acute management of an uncomplicated stroke?
   a) Ensure airway is clear and provide oxygen
   b) Urgent CT/MRI
   c) Rapid reduction of blood pressure if raised
   d) Monitor blood glucose, preventing hypoglycaemia or hyperglycaemia with a sliding scale if diabetic
   e) Thrombolysis if patient in an appropriate centre and fits criteria

8. Which one of the following statements is NOT true of intracranial venous thrombosis (IVT)?
   a) IVT most commonly occurs in the sagittal sinus
   b) Focal symptoms come on within hours
   c) Symptoms include headache, vomiting, seizures and altered vision
   d) Can also manifest as cranial nerve deficits
   e) CT/MRI may show an absent sinus

9. Alzheimer disease does not have which ONE of the following cardinal features?
   a) Visio-spatial impairments, patients often lose their way
   b) Memory loss
   c) Ability to make coherent judgements
   d) Verbal deterioration
   e) Specific cognitive deficiency

10. Which ONE of the following would NOT be seen in the features of a frontal lobe space-occupying lesion?
    a) Double vision
    b) Personality changes
    c) Loss of smell
    d) One-sided weakness
    e) Loss of motivation and ambition

11. Which one of the following treatments is not indicated in the management of myasthenia gravis?
    a) Methotrexate
    b) Gold therapy
    c) Azathioprine
    d) Intravenous immunoglobulin
    e) Thymectomy

12. A patient presents with progressive weakness in both legs. Which ONE of the following symptoms would you NOT expect in suspected cauda equina syndrome?
    a) Nerve root pain at the site of compression
    b) Urinary retention
    c) Constipation
    d) Back pain with radicular pain bilaterally
    e) Areflexia

13. Which ONE of the following statements is not part of the immediate management of subarachnoid haemorrhage (SAH)?
    a) CT within 48 hours of insult, repeated if suspicion of extension
    b) Referral to neurosurgery if proven SAH
    c) Calcium channel blocker treatment to prevent vasospasm
    d) Maintain cerebral perfusion with intravenous fluids
    e) Lumbar puncture within the first 12 hours of insult, prior to CT

14. Which ONE of the following statements is NOT true of multiple sclerosis?
    a) MS is a disease disseminated in time and space; symptoms are relapsing and remitting
    b) There are definitive tests which are pathognomonic for MS
    c) Treatment can be with methylprednisolone, or monoclonal antibodies
    d) Patients usually present with one specific symptom
    e) Symptoms can be stress induced

15. A 42-year-old woman presents with pain in her hand and arm, worse overnight. She is diabetic and has noticed that her palm in the affected hand appears flatter.

What is the most likely diagnosis?

a) Median nerve compression
b) Ulnar nerve compression
c) Radial nerve compression
d) Phrenic nerve compression
e) Tibial nerve compression

Extended matching questions

Question 1
Select one or more options from the list in answer to the questions that follow:
a) Parkinson disease
b) MAO-B inhibitors
c) Delirium
d) Adenosine A2A receptor blockers
e) Anticholinergics
f) Dopamine antagonists
g) Levodopa with dopa-decarboxylase inhibitor
h) Stiffness
i) Hyperkinesia
j) Tremor
k) Micrographia
l) Depression
m) Reduced muscle tone
n) Dementia

1. An 86-year-old man presents with increasing falls, difficulty moving and becoming stuck in a particular position. What THREE other symptoms would you typically expect in this patient?
2. This same patient is likely to need specific treatment for his condition. Which TWO treatments from the list are most likely to be used in the course of this patient's treatment?
3. Which TWO complications from the list would you expect most commonly in this condition?

Question 2
Select one or more options from the list in answer to the questions that follow:
a) Migraine
b) Cluster headaches
c) Tension headache
d) Space-occupying lesion
e) Giant cell arteritis
f) Extradural haemorrhage
g) Meningitis
h) Encephalitis
i) Amitriptyline
j) Verapamil
k) Carbamazepine
l) Cyclizine
m) NSAIDs
n) Sumatriptan
o) Steroids

1. A 43-year-old man presents with a severe unilateral headache and pain in one eye. He has had four similar episodes in the last two weeks. What is the most likely diagnosis and which TWO treatments would you recommend?
2. A 56-year-old man presents with a headache that has been present for a few weeks. The patient also complains of pain in his jaw when chewing. What is the most likely diagnosis and best treatment?
3. A 19-year-old female patient presents with frequent loss of vision on one side of her vision, followed by a headache. Her symptoms are often associated with nausea and vomiting. She presents with active symptoms.

   What is the most likely diagnosis and TWO best treatment options for her headache?

Question 3

Select one or more of the options from the list in answer to the questions that follow:
a) Generalised tonic–clonic seizure
b) Absence seizures
c) Complex partial seizures
d) Myoclonic seizures
e) Akinetic seizures
f) Simple partial seizures
g) Infantile spasms
h) Inform DVLA
i) Allow patient to inform DVLA themselves
j) Carbamazepine
k) Sodium valproate
l) Phenytoin
m) Lamotrigine
n) Vigabatrin
o) Levetiracetam

1. A patient presents with a known diagnosis of epilepsy; she has had primary generalised seizures in the past. Which one type of seizure can lead to unconsciousness?
2. A patient with known epilepsy presents to the GP surgery one month after diagnosis for review and repeat prescription. He has driven to the appointment and advises you he is in a hurry as he needs to return to work.
   You advise him of the implications of his diagnosis and that he should refrain from driving. You note he has been given this information previously from the notes.
   What ONE action do you take?
3. A 32-year-old patient with known partial epilepsy presents to her GP for a repeat prescription of her medication. Which two medications might you expect her to be taking one of?

Answers

Single best answer questions

Q1 d.

An upper motor neurone lesion is as a result of damage to the motor pathways from anywhere between the motor nerve cells in the precentral gyrus to the anterior horn cells in the cord. Hence whole muscle groups are affected as opposed to individual muscles.

An upper motor neurone lesion results in hyperreflexia and hence an upgoing plantar response when eliciting the Babinski sign. The only exception to this is in the initial few hours of an upper motor neurone lesion when it can mimic a lower motor neurone lesion.

Q2 a.

The middle cerebral artery is a branch of the carotid artery and supplies the lateral part of each hemisphere; occlusion of this vessel would result in symptoms on the contralateral aspect of the body and hence a contralateral homonymous hemianopia would develop from damage to the optic radiation.

Q3 e.

Pizotifen is a serotonin antagonist and is typically used in migraine prophylaxis. Sumatriptan and lithium are agonists, and fluoxetine is a specific serotonin reuptake inhibitor. Buspirone is a partial agonist.

Q4 d.

To test the quadriceps femoris, the patient would need to tense the muscle and hence extend the knee; flexing the knee would extend the muscle.

Q5 e.

Purines such as ATP have not as yet been manipulated for any significant clinical conditions. Serotonin receptors are acted on for migraine, depression and psychosis. Adrenaline/noradrenaline receptors are used in asthma, blood pressure, depression, angina and thyroid disease. Acetylcholine receptors are used in treatments for asthma, Parkinson disease and glaucoma. Dopamine receptors are classically used for Parkinson disease medication and in antipsychotics. These lists are not exhaustive but show the relevance of these neurotransmitters.

Q6 e.

In an acute stroke, regardless of whether it is haemorrhagic or embolic, the spasticity develops later. There is initially a flaccid paralysis which then becomes spastic with hyperreflexia.

If the stroke is haemorrhagic the patient may have also complained of severe, sudden-onset headache and meningism and may also progress to a coma.

Q7 c.
Rapid reduction of blood pressure can further exacerbate the damage from the initial stroke as the raised blood pressure is a physiological response to the insult of hypoxia to the brain. Reducing the blood pressure would reduce blood flow to the brain, causing further impairment by preventing autoregulation.

Q8 b.
Intracranial venous thrombosis presents over days and weeks with focal neurological symptoms developing slowly; the only symptom to present early is that of a severe headache.

Treatment following investigation can involve thrombolysis; however, outcomes are variable.

Q9 e.
Alzheimer disease is differentiated from other dementia-causing illnesses by its global effect on the brain. All functions are affected with far-reaching and debilitating effects.

Q10 a.
This deficit would be seen in an occipital lobe lesion. The remaining features could occur as a result of a frontal lobe lesion dependent on where the lesion develops and also the size and rate of growth.

Q11 b.
Methotrexate, prednisolone and azathioprine are used to help suppress the immune system. Intravenous immunoglobulin is used in myasthenic crisis and thymectomy is considered in those patients who are younger and have shown more resistance to less invasive methods.

Q12 a.
Cauda equina syndrome is as a result of cord compression lower down the cord, hence patients experience lower back pain and radicular pain in the legs. Patients with lesions higher in the cord are more likely to have specific nerve root symptoms.

Q13 e.
The lumbar puncture is only carried out in patients in whom radiological investigation is negative, and is usually done after the first 12 hours.

Q14 b.
There is no test as yet which is pathognomonic for MS; symptoms are recorded and evidence of disease dissemination in time and space is needed. Hence the diagnosis is often made over time as more than one event is needed that is not attributable to another cause.

Q15 a.
This is a classic presentation for carpal tunnel syndrome which is a result of reduced space through the wrist for all the necessary structures that pass through it. Patients also complain of paraesthesia in the thumb and some sensory loss. On examination there is often wasting of the thenar eminence, and symptoms can be reproduced by tapping over the wrist (Tinel test).

Extended matching questions
Question 1
Q1 h, j, k.
This patient is presenting with some of the features of Parkinson disease. Along with these features, patients when examined often have a mask-like facies and shuffling gait.

Q2 f, d.
Dopamine agonists are used in Parkinson disease, not antagonists. MAO-B inhibitors can be used in early Parkinson disease, though not when well established. Adenosine receptor blockers are a new, though not established, treatment.

Q3 l, n.
Patients with Parkinson disease are susceptible to both dementia and depression, which are common complications of disease progression. They can also occur as a result of medication side effects. Depression can be treated with SSRIs.

Question 2
Q1 b, j, n.
The diagnosis is cluster headaches as the patient has the classic presentation, which is also often associated with facial flushing, watering and bloodshot eye, and possibly meiosis with ptosis on the affected side.

Patients are treated with sumatriptan as the headache begins and can be given verapamil for prevention.

Q2 e, o.
The patient when examined may have a thickened tender temporal artery; the pain on chewing is likely to be as a result of jaw claudication.

Q3 a, m, n.
The patient has the classic presentation of migrainous headache preceded by visual aura. The two best treatments are NSAIDs and triptan therapy which have been shown to have similar efficacy.

The patient may also be prescribed later with prophylactic treatment to prevent further attacks.

Question 3

Q1 a.

Generalised tonic–clonic seizures can result in loss of consciousness and post-ictal confusion and drowsiness. Patients may also experience Todd paralysis where they have partial or complete paralysis of the body for a period of time after the seizure. This resolves completely.

Q2 h.

The patient has been advised that he should refrain from driving but has refused to do this. As a clinician there is a duty of care to report him to the DVLA to ensure that he does not put others at risk. Patients can reapply to the DVLA for permission to drive a car once they have been completely seizure-free for 1 year.

Q3 k or m.

These two medications are the best two options for partial epilepsy. Most patients' epilepsy can be controlled with one agent, though occasionally two agents are used.

12 Ophthalmology

For each question below, what is the most likely answer?
Select one or more options from the answers supplied.

1. At what distance should a Snellen chart be read?
   a) 1 metre
   b) 2 metres
   c) 6 metres
   d) 6 feet
   e) 12 feet

2. Hyperthyroidism is associated with which one of the following?
   a) Ectropian
   b) Entropian
   c) Blepharitis
   d) Xanthelasma
   e) Exophthalmos

3. Which one of the following is, worldwide, the most common cause of blindness?
   a) Cataract
   b) Glaucoma
   c) Vitamin A deficiency
   d) Tracoma
   e) Onchocerciasis

4. Which of the following is NOT a malignant lesion of the eyelid?
   a) Squamous cell carcinoma
   b) Malignant melanoma
   c) Basal cell carcinoma
   d) Keratoacanthoma
   e) Karposi sarcoma

The Complete GPVTS Stage 2 Preparation Guide: Questions and Professional Dilemmas,
First Edition. Edited by Saba Khan with Neel Sharma.
© 2012 John Wiley & Sons, Ltd. Published 2012 by John Wiley & Sons, Ltd.

5. Which one of the following causes of red eye requires no treatment?
   a) Scleritis
   b) Anterior uveitis
   c) Acute closed-angle glaucoma
   d) Subconjunctival haemorrhage
   e) Episcleritis

6. Which one of the following is NOT a treatment for acute closed-angle glaucoma?
   a) Alpha-adrenergic agonists
   b) Beta-blockers
   c) Peripheral iridectomy
   d) Cyclopentolate
   e) Prostaglandin analogues

7. Which of the following causes sudden painless loss of vision?
   a) Cataract
   b) Central retinal vein occlusion
   c) Central retinal artery occlusion
   d) Macular degeneration
   e) Retinal detachment

8. Which single answer is NOT associated with Horner syndrome?
   a) Multiple sclerosis
   b) Pancoast tumour
   c) Posterior inferior cerebellar artery occlusion
   d) Aortic aneurysm
   e) Addison's disease

9. Acute closed-angle glaucoma presents with which single feature?
   a) Reduced pupil size
   b) No change in visual acuity
   c) Photophobia
   d) Severe pain
   e) Normal corneal appearance

10. Which single answer is the best treatment for kerato-conjunctivitis sicca?
   a) Steroid drops
   b) Topical acyclovir
   c) Chloramphenicol
   d) Artificial tears
   e) Laser treatment

11. Which multi-system disorder has no eye manifestations?
   a) Wilson disease
   b) Hyperthyroidism
   c) Hypoparathyroidism

d) Dermatomyositis

e) Gout

12. Which two of the following cranial nerves are associated with eye movements?

a) Third cranial nerve

b) Fifth cranial nerve

c) Sixth cranial nerve

d) Seventh cranial nerve

e) Tenth cranial nerve

13. Which treatment is best for allergic conjunctivitis?

a) Oral steroids

b) Oral antihistamines

c) Topical antihistamine drops

d) Hypromellose drops

e) Steroid drops

14. Which single statement is true of age-related macular degeneration?

a) Bitemporal hemianopia is a feature

b) Central visual loss occurs

c) Complete blindness is inevitable

d) Short sightedness

e) Is reversible with prompt treatment

15. Which of these conditions do NOT cause floaters?

a) Retinal detachment

b) Recurrent vitreous bleeding

c) Diabetic retinopathy

d) Tuberculosis

e) Glaucoma

Extended matching questions

Question 1
Choose the single most appropriate answer for the following questions from the list provided.
a) Choroid melanoma
b) Dry age-related macular degeneration
c) Optic atrophy
d) Retinal artery occlusion
e) Vitreous haemorrhage
f) Anterior ischaemic optic neuropathy
g) Wet age-related macular degeneration
h) Retinal artery vein occlusion
i) Branch retinal vein occlusion
j) Choroiditis
k) Tobacco-alcohol amblyopia
l) Cataract

1. A 79-year-old man presents with a gradual deterioration of vision. Examination reveals drusen and degenerative change at the macula, with little choroidal new vessel formation. What is the diagnosis?
2. A 63-year-old woman with chronic ischaemic heart disease presents with sudden dramatic loss of vision in one eye; her visual acuity has been reduced to finger counting. What is the most likely diagnosis?
3. A 50-year-old man who has a history of liver disease, and ischaemic heart disease, presents with a history of loss of red/green discrimination followed by gradual loss of vision. What is the most likely diagnosis?

Question 2
From the list below, choose the single best answer for the following clinical scenarios:
a) Cataract
b) Retinal detachment
c) Macular holes
d) Retinal detachment
e) Vascular retinopathy
f) Microaneurysms
g) Nystagmus
h) Pseudopapilloedema
i) Retinitis pigmentosa
j) Trachoma
k) Toxoplasm
l) Diabetic retinopathy
m) Papilloedema

1. A 48-year-old woman is found to have hard exudates, macular oedema, haemorrhages and papilloedema. There are also some flame haemorrhages with cottonwool spots as well as 'silver wiring' of the arterioles. What is the diagnosis?
2. A young woman is diagnosed with raised intracranial pressure; she is found to have bilateral disc changes showing swollen discs, hidden disc margins, congested retinal veins and a few haemorrhages. Which condition best describes these changes?
3. A 60-year-old man presents with symptoms of a 'curtain falling down over his eyes'; he has no pain and when questioned further describes flashing lights, floaters and reduced visual acuity. What is the most likely diagnosis?

Question 3

From the list below, choose the single best answer for the following scenarios:

a) Timolol
b) Latanoprost
c) Pilocarpine
d) Brimonidine
e) Acetozolamide
f) Dipivefrine
g) Triamcinolone
h) Ranibizumab
i) Prednisolone
j) Chloramphenicol
k) Acyclovir
l) Ciprofloxacin
m) Sodium cromoglycate
n) Cyclopentolate

1. A patient presents to the Emergency Department in the middle of the night with blurred vision, and seeing haloes around lights. He has severe pain with vomiting, and when examined appears to have a fixed dilated pupil. The eye feels hard when examined. What is the first-line drug treatment in this patient?
2. A 50-year-old man presents with an acutely painful eye, photophobia, blurred vision, lacrimation and a small pupil. Most markedly there is circumcorneal redness. He was recently diagnosed with ankylosing spondylitis. When examined his pain worsens on convergence of the eyes. He is referred to an ophthalmologist. What is the first line of treatment?
3. A 21-year-old man presents with bilateral itchy inflamed conjunctiva. He has a history of asthma and eczema. He does not have any pain, and when examined there is no change to acuity or papillary response. What is the best management for this patient?

Answers

Single best answer questions

Q1 c.
The Snellen chart is used to measure visual acuity in each eye by sitting the patient 6 metres away from the chart and asking them to read the row of letters as far down the chart as possible, covering first one eye and then the other. This enables the Snellen fraction (6/x) to be determined for each eye, where x (the row identifier) is the distance at which this size of type is normally visible. This is a simple and useful measure that can be used in short consultations to assess visual acuity where needed.

Q2 e.
Graves disease is caused by an autoimmune response that results in hyper-stimulation of the thyroid-stimulating hormone (TSH) receptor. It is also directed at the soft tissues within the orbit; the typical appearance of protruding eyes is as a result of increased oedema and inflammation.

Q3 a.
Blindness around the world is more common in developing countries and hence causes in these parts of the world are more significant. Cataract and glaucoma are still the biggest causes with onchocerciasis being the next most common cause.

Blindness is classified as acute or gradual onset and then as bilateral or unilateral. Any patient with sudden visual loss should have a secondary care review.

Q4 d.
Keratoacanthoma is a benign skin lesion that is made up of a central keratin-filled cavity surrounded by a symmetrical border of epidermis. The lesion is self-limiting and, if left untreated, will usually resolve within two months. Surgery is only indicated if there is histological confusion or if there is atrophic scarring left behind.

Q5 d.
Subconjunctival haemorrhage, though dramatic in appearance, does not need any further referral or management. Most patients can be reassured and advised that it will resolve. The blood is usually as a result of rupture of a small vessel; this can be due to trauma, coughing or hypertension. If recurrent then patients should have their blood pressure checked and also clotting studies done.

Q6 d.
Cyclopentolate is a mydriatic, and in this case would worsen acute closed-angle glaucoma. In this condition part of the treatment is to constrict the pupil with topical pilocarpine, to allow drainage of the canal of

Schlemm. Patients should be referred urgently and are given intravenous acetozolamide to reduce intraocular pressure.

Q7 b, c, e.
Acute loss of vision in any patient should be referred to secondary care for review. Those with bilateral loss are investigated for stroke, papilloedema and methyl alcohol poisoning. If it is unilateral sudden blindness then patients would be managed for possible central retinal vein/artery occlusion, vitreous haemorrhage, temporal arteritis, retinal detachment or optic neuritis dependent on the history and presenting features.

Q8 e.
Horner syndrome comprises of ptosis, miosis and ipsilateral anhydrosis. It is as a result of interruption of the sympathetic nerves from the hypothalamus to the orbit. The cause can be central or peripheral with central causes including vascular accidents, demyelination or tumours. Peripheral causes include apical lung disease, thyroid enlargement and neck trauma.

Q9 d.
A typical case of acute closed-angle glaucoma would present as a patient with loss of vision in the affected eye. There is often severe pain with nausea and vomiting. When examined the patient will have a hardened globe, marked redness of the sclera, and a non-reactive semi-dilated pupil. The cornea has a hazy corneal reflex.

Q10 d.
Kerato-conjunctivitis sicca is a condition which results in dry eyes, as a result of reduced lacrimal duct secretions. Patients complain of dryness of the eyes with some discomfort, which worsens during the day with itchiness. The diagnosis can be confirmed with the Schirmer test. This involves placing a small piece of absorbent paper against the lower fornix; for a negative diagnosis the length of paper wetted in 5 minutes must exceed 10 mm. This condition is part of Sjögren syndrome, and is found in systemic lupus erythematosus and sarcoidosis.

Q11 d.
Wilson disease is associated with Kayser–Fleischer rings, which are deposits of copper around the corneal border, which appear as a brownish discoloration. Hyperthyroidism can be as a result of Graves disease which specifically targets the eyes, resulting in proptosis, ophthalmoplegia and papilloedema. Hypoparathyroidism is associated with cataract formation and patients with gout can develop sore eyes as a result of monosodium urate deposition in the conjunctiva.

Dermatomyositis is a condition affecting the muscles, where muscle biopsy shows rhabdomyolysis. The cause is unknown though some drugs have been implicated.

Q12 a, c.
The third cranial nerve innervates all the muscles controlling the eye except for the lateral rectus which is the sixth cranial nerve and the superior oblique which is the fourth. The oculomotor nerve also carries the parasympathetic supply which constricts the pupil.

Q13 c.
Allergic conjunctivitis presents with seasonal symptoms of itching, conjunctival oedema and mild redness of the eyes. It is best treated with topical antihistamines and avoidance of the allergen, if known.

Q14 b.
Age-related macular degeneration occurs in patients over 50 with changes to the macula, specifically the presence of drusens which are lipid and protein deposits. Patients develop progressive loss of their central vision as the macula degenerates. Peripheral vision can be maintained.

Q15 e.
Floaters are dark spots that move within the visual field while the eye is at rest; they can result from degenerative opacities in the vitreous. Patients should be examined before reassuring to ensure there is no retinal disease or vitreous change. Patients who have sudden showers of floaters need urgent referral as this could be secondary to a bleed from a retinal detachment.

Extended matching questions
Question 1
Q1 b.
Dry age-related macular degeneration is associated with increasing age and damage to the macula. The patient notices loss of central vision with sparing of the periphery. There is no pain associated with this condition, and symptoms are usually bilateral.

Wet age-related macular degeneration is characterised by a similar clinical presentation but when examined the eyes have choroidal neovascular lesions. These vessels leak, causing haemorrhage within the structures of the eye followed by scar formation that impairs vision further. Dry age-related macular degeneration is treated with counselling and rehabiliatation. However, if patients are suspected of having wet age-related macular degeneration, then urgent referral is required for assessment for one of the following treatments:

- laser photocoagulation
- photodynamic therapy with verteporfin
- anti-angiogenic therapy

Q2 d.

Retinal artery occlusion can be as a result of emboli, thrombus or vasospasm. Patients present with sudden dramatic painless loss of vision. When examined the patients have a poor or non-existent papillary response in the affected eye. The retina appears pale and opaque with thin thread arteries, the fovea remains vascularised, hence the 'cherry red spot appearance'.

Sudden loss of vision is an ophthalmological emergency and requires immediate referral. Blood testing may reveal a high ESR indicating giant cell arteritis.

Patients are treated with rapid reduction in intraocular pressure to promote blood flow, and dislodge clot or emboli. This can be done by massage of the globe, intravenous acetozolamide or paracentesis.

Q3 k.

Tobacco-alcohol amblyopia is a condition of poor nutrition and toxin-mediated damage. Thiamine deficiency and some of the toxins from cigarettes are some of the causative factors.

The condition leads to central loss of vision followed by loss of green, then red and, if severe, white. Patients can be treated with thiamine, vitamin B12, folate and removal of toxic agents. Some reversal of the damage caused can be achieved.

Question 2

Q1 e.

Vascular retinopathy can occur in patients with hypertension. The changes described are typical for patients with uncontrolled hypertension. With adequate blood pressure control, haemorrhages and cottonwool spots can clear, though hard exudates can take longer. Papilloedema will also resolve though this can remain and also lead to optic atrophy, affecting vision more seriously.

Q2 m.

Papilloedema is essentially congestion of the optic disc as a result of raised intracranial pressure. Intracranial pressure can be raised as a result of any number of causes, with patients presenting with headache, vomiting, disturbed vision and reduced level of consciousness if severe.

If patients present with papilloedema with neurological signs or symptoms, then urgent referral may be required where a potential brain tumour is suspected. Symptoms may include seizures, nerve palsies, severe headaches and altered cognitive or mental states.

Q3 d.

Retinal detachment occurs when fluid accumulates in the subretinal space, or from traction secondary to scarring. The retina may also detach as a result of trauma on the myopic eye, which becomes elongated.

These patients will present with sudden loss of vision and hence need urgent referral to secondary care. If patients are seen quickly enough, they can have surgery to repair the detachment or tear, and preserve the blood supply to the macula and hence conserve vision.

Question 3

Q1 c.

The clinical scenario described is typical of acute closed-angle glaucoma. These patients need urgent referral to secondary care. Patients are treated with pilocarpine to constrict the pupil and unblock the canal of Schlemm, allowing drainage of fluid and relieving the condition. They are also treated with intravenous acetozolamide when in secondary care to reduce intraocular pressure. Surgical treatment may be an option in patients where medical treatment fails.

Q2 i.

This clinical scenario describes acute iritis, which is associated with patients suffering from ankylosing spondylitis. Iritis is essentially inflammation of the anterior part of the uvea. Patients should be referred to hospital, and are treated dependent on the cause. If an infective cause is suspected, appropriate antiviral/antibiotic treatment will be given. Analgesia and mydriatics are given to reduce pain and prevent ciliary spasm. Prednisolone is used to suppress inflammation and surgical causes are looked for and treated as appropriate.

Q3 m.

This patient has an allergic conjunctivitis, this characteristically affects both eyes and can be intensely itchy. It is usually seasonal and is associated with hayfever.

Patients can manifest symptoms from a very young age, and can be affected quite severely, resulting in absence from school. Boys are more commonly affected, and symptoms are more intense at the pubertal stage.

When examined, patients have the typical cobblestone appearance from papillary proliferation. Treatment is with topical sodium cromoglycate drops, which is usually long term.

13 Paediatrics

For each question below, what is the most likely answer?
Select ONE option only from the answers supplied.

1. You are an F2 doctor working in general practice. Your first patient is a
   15-month-old boy accompanied by his mother. You see from his notes
   that he has not yet received his MMR immunisation. You ask the
   mother about this and she tells you the MMR vaccine has been shown
   to cause autism. What is your response to her statement?
   a) Advise her that her child should have the MMR anyway as there is
      only a weak link between MMR and autism.
   b) State that there is absolutely no link between MMR and autism and
      that her son would be at risk of measles, mumps and rubella if not
      given the vaccine.
   c) State that if she is concerned, her son could have the measles,
      mumps and rubella vaccinations separately.
   d) State that ultimately it is her decision and she is responsible for her
      child.
   e) State that these diseases are uncommon and her son should be
      protected by herd immunity.

2. You are an F2 doctor working in the paediatric Emergency Department.
   A 3-year-old child comes in with a presumed febrile seizure. Which of
   the following is NOT consistent with a febrile seizure?
   a) A seizure triggered by a fever associated with an upper respiratory
      tract infection
   b) The absence of focal neurology
   c) A normally developing child between 6 months and 5 years with no
      past medical history
   d) A duration of less than 5 minutes
   e) The presence of myoclonic jerk

The Complete GPVTS Stage 2 Preparation Guide: Questions and Professional Dilemmas,
First Edition. Edited by Saba Khan with Neel Sharma.
© 2012 John Wiley & Sons, Ltd. Published 2012 by John Wiley & Sons, Ltd.

3. You are an F2 doctor working in general practice. Your first patient is a 5-year-old girl with mild flexural eczema. Which regime would you prescribe?
   a) Emollients, soap substitutes and hydrocortisone when needed
   b) Emollients and a short course of Betnovate for the affected areas
   c) Emollients and Trimovate cream

4. You are an F2 doctor working in a paediatric ward. A 4-year-old patient is admitted with dehydration due to a diarrhoeal illness. What is you first-line diagnostic investigation?
   a) Stool culture for ova, cysts and parasites
   b) A blood culture
   c) An abdominal X-ray
   d) A full blood count
   e) Urea and electrolytes

5. Which of the following is NOT indicative of non-accidental injury?
   a) Fingertip bruising
   b) Torn frenulum
   c) Flexural eczema

6. What is the most likely diagnosis in a child who presents with a week's history of fever, red eyes, peeling skin and swelling of the hands and feet, rash and lymphadenopathy?
   a) Kawasaki disease
   b) Conjunctivitis
   c) Upper respiratory tract infection
   d) Meningitis

7. Which is the gold standard investigation for gastro-oesophageal reflux?
   a) Barium swallow
   b) Nuclear medicine milk scan
   c) pH study
   d) Upper gastrointestinal endoscopy

8. You are an F2 doctor working in general practice. You see a 2-month-old girl with a history suggestive of functional reflux. She is otherwise well and is following her centiles. What is your initial management plan?
   a) Arrange some investigations to confirm the cause
   b) Advise the mother on feeding practice and posture and organise a review appointment
   c) Start a proton pump inhibitor

9. Which of the following are NOT typical features of gastro-oesophageal reflux disease?
   a) Irritability with feeds
   b) Excessive vomiting
   c) Excessive hiccups
   d) Generalised irritability
   e) Failure to thrive

10. Which of the following is a cause of failure to thrive?
    a) Coeliac disease
    b) Cows' milk protein intolerance
    c) Recurrent urinary tract infection
    d) Gastro-oesophageal reflux
    e) All of the above

11. You are an F2 doctor working in the paediatric Emergency Department. You see an 8-year-old with anaphylaxis. Which dose of adrenaline should be given?
    a) 0.25 mL of 1:10 000 solution
    b) 0.25 mL of 1:100 000 solution
    c) 0.5 mL of 1:1000 solution
    d) 0.25 mL of 1:1000 solution

12. An 8-year-old child is admitted with an asthma attack. Which feature(s) would indicate life-threatening asthma?
    a) A wheezy child who is able to talk
    b) Oxygen saturation of less than 92% in an agitated child
    c) A heart rate of more than 120 beats per minute
    d) A peak flow rate of 40% of predicted
    e) A respiratory rate of more than 30 breaths per minute

13. You are an F2 doctor working in general practice. You see a 5-year-old girl with an itchy scalp. She says her friend at school was also itching. On examination, you see small white dots attached to her hair. What is your diagnosis and management?
    a) Psoriasis: you prescribe a scalp steroid solution
    b) Scabies: you prescribe malathion and advise wet combing
    c) Headlice: you prescribe malathion and advise wet combing

14. What are the advantages of breast feeding?
    a) Reduced gut and respiratory infections
    b) Encourages maternal bonding
    c) Cheap and convenient
    d) It is a protective factor against breast cancer in the mother
    e) All of the above

15. You are an F2 doctor working in general practice. You take a call from a patient who is calling for advice. She is a new mother and was discharged from hospital 8 hours after an uncomplicated normal vaginal delivery early this morning. She has noticed that her newborn baby is yellow. What is your course of action?
    a) Arrange an immediate referral to hospital
    b) State that it is probably breast milk jaundice and arrange for her to be reviewed in the practice in a few days
    c) Arrange a health visitor visit

Extended matching questions

Question 1
For each of the following scenarios select the SINGLE best answer for the most likely diagnosis, from the list below:
a) Slipped upper epiphysis
b) Transient synovitis
c) Juvenile arthritis
d) Rheumatoid arthritis
e) Meningococcal septicaemia
f) Septic arthritis
j) Henoch–Schönlein purpura
k) Growing pains
l) Non-accidental injury
m) Congenital dislocation of the hip
n) Idiopathic musculoskeletal pain
o) Perthes disease

1. Your patient is a 7-year-old girl with a limp. She denies a history of trauma, feels well in herself and states that she woke up with left hip pain. What is the most likely diagnosis?
2. Your patient is a 2-year-old girl who refuses to walk. She has a fever and screams if carried. Her mother noticed her hip felt warm when she changed her nappy. What is the most likely diagnosis?
3. Your patient is a 6-year-old boy with a 3-week history of limp and right hip pain. He is well in himself but he has limited hip movements when you examine him. What is the most likely diagnosis?
4. The nurse asks you to review a 6-month-old baby after her vaccinations. She attended the surgery with her uncle and was 2 months overdue for her vaccinations. She was irritable when lifted and if her hip was moved. She is apyrexial. On examination, you notice several small bruises over her hip. What is the most likely diagnosis?

Question 2
For each of the following scenarios select the SINGLE best answer for the most likely diagnosis, from the list below:
a) Tonsillitis
b) Whooping cough
c) Viral pneumonia
d) Asthma
e) Gastro-oesophageal reflux
f) Tuberculosis
g) Acute bronchitis
h) Viral-induced wheeze
i) Bacterial pneumonia
j) Allergy
k) Bronchiolitis

l) Cystic fibrosis
m) Viral upper respiratory tract infection
n) Epiglottitis
o) Croup

1. Your patient is a 5-year-old boy with a 4-month history of episodic noisy breathing and cough, especially in the early morning. It is worse when he visits his grandparents who live on a farm. He is otherwise well. What condition is he most likely to be suffering from?
2. Your patient is a 3-year-old boy with a 2-day history of a barking cough and temperature of 38.2°C. His mother has noticed he makes strange sounds when he breathes in. What is the most likely diagnosis?
3. Your patient is a 10-month-old girl with coryzal symptoms and cough. Her mother is worried as she is sometimes too breathless to feed. She is apyrexial and on chest examination you hear a high-pitched wheeze and widespread crepitations over her lung fields. What condition is she likely to have?
4. Your patient is a 6-year-old boy with a runny nose, sore throat and occasional cough. He was running around in the reception room when you called him in. Examination is normal. What is the diagnosis?

Question 3
For each of the following scenarios select the SINGLE best answer for the most suitable first-line treatment, from the list below:
a) Erythromycin
b) Malathion
c) Emollients and hydrocortisone 1%
d) Aciclovir
e) Intramuscular benzylpenicillin
f) Oral penicillin V
g) Emollients and Betnovate cream
h) Emollients
i) Hydrocortisone
j) Clotrimazole
k) Eumovate
l) Fucidin
m) Trimovate
n) Antihistamines
o) Oral flucloxacillin

1. Your patient is a 15-month-old boy with a dry red rash on his face, scalp and flexures. His mother feels it has worsened in the last 3 months. Which option would you pick for treatment?
2. Your patient is a 3-year-old girl with three episodes of transient red itchy swellings of the skin. They usually last minutes to an hour and resolve. The skin then looks normal. How would you manage this?

3. Your patient is a 2-year-old boy who has been increasingly irritable over the last few hours. His mother reports he had a cold yesterday but today is feverish, off his food and drowsy. She noticed his feet feel cold and he has a rash. What is the first line management?

4. Your patient is a 5-year-old girl who has just started school and has developed small red spots on her face. On examination, they have a yellow crust and look like blisters and are spreading to her chest. She is otherwise systemically well. Her younger sibling has a similar rash. What is the most likely diagnosis?

Answers

Single best answer questions

Q1 b.

Huge controversy surrounded the safety of the MMR vaccine. The theory that linked the MMR vaccine to autism and Crohn disease has been widely discredited. The MMR vaccine is given at 13 months with a second dose at 3–5 years. Measles can cause otitis media, pneumonia, fits and encephalitis and can be fatal. Mumps can cause pancreatitis, meningitis and can result in deafness. In boys, it can cause orchitis and lead to infertility. Rubella or German measles is usually a mild illness, although can cause fetal abnormalities if contracted during the first 20 weeks of pregnancy.

Q2 e.

A myoclonic fit is indicative of epilepsy. Febrile seizures are common and are diagnosed by answers a) to d) and occur as the temperature rises during a febrile illness. Parent education and reassurance are key. Tepid sponging, fever management and diazepam per rectum can be used if prolonged.

Q3 a.

The mainstay of management of mild flexural ezcema is emollients. Parent and patient education is crucial. If needed, a mild steroid can be used and, if response is inadequate, a moderate-potency steroid can be used for short duration.

Q4 a.

Although viral gastroenteritis is the most common scenario and rotavirus the most common cause, it is important to exclude other causes of diarrhea, especially if there is a significant travel history, although this is not mentioned here. Bacterial causes include *Campylobacter, Staphylococcus, E. coli* and *Salmonella*. Blood tests would be helpful, especially to assess the extent of dehydration.

Q5 c.

A torn tongue frenulum is indicative of shaking and may be associated with vitreous or retinal bleeds. Abuse may be physical, emotional, sexual or by neglect. Risk factors include a low birthweight baby, a young mother, stress, lower socioeconomic classes and unwanted pregnancy. Suspect abuse if disclosed by the child, there is an odd mode of injury, inconsistent history, late presentation, avoidance of full physical examination. In addition, an unexplained fracture or injury to buttocks, perineum or face should raise the alert.

Q6 a.

There is no specific diagnostic test for Kawasaki disease, therefore diagnosis is based on clinical grounds, i.e. fever of 5 days' duration plus four of the following five criteria: conjunctival injection, lymphadenopathy, rash, changes in extremities or changes in lips or oral mucosa. Alternatively, the presence of fever and coronary artery aneurysms with three additional criteria are diagnostic. The treatment is with aspirin and intravenous immunoglobulin, and is aimed at reducing inflammation and preventing the occurrence of coronary artery aneurysms.

Q7 c.
These are all possible investigations but their use depends on the clinical picture and severity. Barium radiology will pick up anatomical problems such as malrotation or stricture. Nuclear medicine 'milk' scan will assess acid or alkali reflux following a physiological meal and assess gastric emptying. Endoscopy requires inpatient admission in infants and children and is not a first-line procedure.

Q8 b.
Functional reflux is very common and does not usually require specific treatment. Initial discussion should centre around parental education and review of feeding practices such as excessive feeding, frequent feeds and posture. Milk thickeners can be used. Specific treatments include acid suppressants such as ranitidine or omeprazole, and prokinetic drugs such as domperidone.

Q9 d.
Gastro-oesophageal reflux is very common in infancy and is due to an immature lower oesophageal sphincter. Irritability is common when associated with feeds which may also cause arching and food refusal. Generalised irritability is an atypical feature and other causes should be considered.

Q10 e.
These are all organic causes for failure to thrive, which is a failure to gain weight at an adequate rate. A full history and examination are essential to ascertain whether due to organic causes. The management of non-organic failure to thrive may involve the health visitor.

Q11 d.
For an adult or child over 12 years the dose is 0.5 mL adrenaline 1:1000 solution. In children aged 6–12 years it is half the adult dose. This dose is repeated if improvement is transient or there is no improvement or if the child deteriorates after initial assessment. Anaphylaxis is a severe systemic allergic reaction and common causes include food (nuts, fish, sesame seeds, milk, eggs), wasp or bee stings and drugs such as antibiotics.

Q12 b.
Answers c) to e) indicate severe asthma. If the child is able to talk this signifies a moderate asthma exacerbation.

Q13 c.
Headlice are very common, especially in school-aged children. They are contagious and contact tracing is important. An alternative to malathion is permethrin and treatment should be repeated after 7 days.

Q14 e.
Breast feeding should be encourage and mothers should be supported by all healthcare professionals including midwives, health visitors, practice nurses and GPs to address any problems or concerns.

Q15 a.
Any jaundice in the first 24 hours after birth is assumed to be pathological and needs to be investigated immediately. The main causes are infection or haemolysis. Management involves phototherapy and treating the underlying cause.

Extended matching questions
Question 1
Q1 b.
Transient synovitis of the hip or irritable hip. This is the most common cause of a limp in childhood. It usually affects children aged 2–10 years, and the child is systemically well. The cause is unknown and it usually resolves spontaneously after 7–10 days. It is important to exclude other pathology.

Q2 f.
Septic arthritis. This must always be excluded and is an orthopaedic emergency. A systemically unwell child with a hot swollen joint must be admitted. In young children a hip ultrasound is the investigation of choice. Treatment is with intravenous antibiotics.

Q3 o.
Perthes disease is due to avascular necrosis of the femoral head and usually has a gradual onset (unlike scenario 1). Management involves X-ray, orthopaedic referral and may involve bracing or surgery if severe. Recovery is over 2–3 years.

Q4 l.
This should always be a consideration. Fingertip bruising is a tell-tale sign and any bruising in non-mobile babies should raise suspicion. Septic arthritis should be excluded but in this scenario there are several risk factors for non-accidental injury. She is not accompanied by a parent, she is late for her vaccinations and the child presented for another reason.

Question 2
Q1 d.
Childhood asthma affects about 5% of children in the UK. Typical features include wheezing, cough and breathlessness. A detailed history is needed

to determine the pattern of symptoms, especially if there is diurnal variation, triggers and severity of attacks. It is also important to quantify the effect of symptoms on daily activities, school, sport and sleep.

Q2 o.
Croup is a viral infection characterised by a barking cough and inspiratory stridor. Management depends on severity.

Q3 k.
Bronchiolitis peaks in winter months and is caused by respiratory syncitial virus. It usually affects infants and management depends on severity.

Q4 m.
Viral upper respiratory tract infections are very common.

Question 3
Q1 c.
This child has atopic eczema. It affects 10–20% of children and there is usually a family history of atopy. The onset is usually in the first 6 months of life and it can affect the face, scalp and flexures; extensor aspects can also be involved. The mainstay of treatment is parental education, emollients and steroids. In severe or non-responsive cases referral to a dermatologist is indicated.

Q2 n.
This history describes urticaria which can be caused by infection, food, drugs and physical agents but is commonly idiopathic. A good history is essential with detailed trigger factors. Difficulty in swallowing, shortness of breath, drowsiness or feeling unwell should alert you to possible anaphylaxis and needs urgent admission.

Q3 e.
This is meningococcal septicaemia until proven otherwise and is a medical emergency. This child must be transferred immediately to hospital and be given intramuscular benzylpenicillin while waiting for the ambulance.

Q4 o.
This child has impetigo and should be treated with oral antibiotics. This is a superficially spreading skin infection caused by *Staphylococcus aureus* or group A beta-haemolytic streptococcus. If only a few lesions are present, treatment may initially consist of a topical antibacterial cream such as Fucidin.

14 Psychiatry

For each question below, what is the most likely answer?
Select one or more options from the answers supplied.

1. Which single option is the most effective measure for anxiety disorder on its own?
   a) Exercise
   b) Counselling
   c) Cognitive behavioural therapy
   d) Meditation
   e) Benzodiazepines

2. Which ONE of the following is NOT a feature of anorexia nervosa?
   a) BMI 18–20
   b) Thoughts of being overweight despite being thin
   c) Amenorrhoea
   d) Reduced libido (in men)
   e) Fear of weight gain

3. Which ONE of the following features is NOT seen in bipolar disorder?
   a) Pressure of speech
   b) Ideas of grandeur
   c) Increased libido
   d) Increased sleep
   e) Increased irritability

4. Which ONE of the following is NOT an antenatal factor in birth-related mental retardation?
   a) Alcohol
   b) Growth retardation related to nutrition
   c) Infection
   d) Hyperthyroidism
   e) Trauma

The Complete GPVTS Stage 2 Preparation Guide: Questions and Professional Dilemmas,
First Edition. Edited by Saba Khan with Neel Sharma.
© 2012 John Wiley & Sons, Ltd. Published 2012 by John Wiley & Sons, Ltd.

5. Which one of the following features would you NOT expect to see in an adolescent with depression?
   a) Running away
   b) Complaints of boredom
   c) Psychomotor retardation
   d) Antisocial behaviour
   e) Hypersomnia

6. A patient presents with a history of displaying the personality traits of envy, lack of empathy, entitlement, and is arrogant when interacting with people. He also often exploits people and scenarios to exaggerate his own achievements.
   Which ONE of the following personality disorders would this most fit with?
   a) Histrionic
   b) Depressive
   c) Narcissistic
   d) Psychopathic
   e) Schizoid

7. A 79-year-old woman presents with a 3-day history of confusion, disorientation and appears drowsy. She also smells strongly of urine. A urine dipstick test is positive for infection.
   From the following options pick the most likely diagnosis and best single treatment.
   a) Dementia
   b) Delirium
   c) Antibiotics
   d) Haloperidol
   e) Diazepam

8. A 21-year-old girl presents with a normal BMI, complaining of discomfort in her face and on examination you notice calluses on her hands.
   What is the most likely diagnosis?
   a) Anorexia nervosa
   b) Bulimia
   c) Body image disorder
   d) Histrionic personality disorder
   e) Depression

9. A 42-year-old man presents to his GP stating that his neighbour has put a voice into his head to control him.
   Which one of the following best describes his symptoms?
   a) Delusion
   b) Auditory hallucination
   c) Auditory hallucination plus delusion
   d) Obsessional thought plus hallucination
   e) Obsessional thought plus delusion

10. A 23-year-old woman presents to her GP worried as she feels she is becoming more and more fearful of spiders. She finds it is now stopping her from engaging in normal social activities. Which one of the following behavioural therapy options would be best for her?
    a) Response prevention
    b) Systematic desensitisation
    c) Covert conditioning
    d) Social skills training
    e) Positive behaviour support

11. An 8-year-old boy is seen in the paediatric outpatients clinic. He has recently been diagnosed with autism. The family have returned for more explanation of their son's condition.
    Which one of the following symptoms is NOT typical of his condition?
    a) Unaware of the feelings in others
    b) Lack of empathy
    c) Unusual attachments to certain toys
    d) Prefer to have chaotic routines
    e) Avoidance of eye contact

12. Which TWO of the following statements is INCORRECT in relation to the Mental Health Act (MHA) (2007)?
    a) The decision to detain for further assessment under the MHA must be made by at least two doctors and a trained psychiatric nurse.
    b) The decision to detain for further assessment under the MHA must be made by at least two doctors and a social worker (or other trained mental health professional).
    c) The decision to detain under the MHA is reached if the patient is deemed to be a risk to themselves or others unless given urgent treatment from psychiatric services.
    d) The initial period of assessment under the MHA is 28 days.
    e) The initial period of assessment under the MHA is 5 days.

13. Which ONE of the following conditions does NOT have a genetic component?
    a) Alcoholism
    b) Bipolar disorder
    c) Schizophrenia
    d) Autism
    e) Obsessive-compulsive disorder

14. Which of the following is a feature of school refusal?
    a) Truancy
    b) Low social class
    c) Emotional overprotection
    d) School work of a poor standard
    e) Relaxed parenting style

15. Which of the following is true of ADHD?
    a) Diagnosis is usually made as a toddler
    b) Usually persists into adulthood
    c) Diagnostic testing is freely available
    d) More frequent in learning disabled children
    e) Those affected have a lower risk of deliberate self-harm and suicide

16. Night terrors are best related to which of the following?
    a) 55% of children experience night terrors
    b) Most common between ages 2–6
    c) Can only occur under the age of 12
    d) Last over 1 hour
    e) Resolve quicker if a child psychologist is involved

Extended matching questions

Question 1
Select one or more of the following options in answer to the following questions:
a) Hypnagogic hallucinations
b) Auditory hallucination in the third person
c) Tactile hallucination
d) Primary delusions
e) Visual hallucinations
f) Secondary delusions
g) Obsessional thoughts
h) Thought insertion
i) Oral olanzapine
j) Intramuscular haloperidol
k) Oral lorazepam
l) Intramuscular procyclidine
m) Chlorpromazine
n) Quetiapine

1. Which THREE of the above symptoms on their own would be sufficient for a diagnosis of schizophrenia?
2. Which TWO of the above symptoms would be considered NOT part of any psychiatric condition?
3. Which TWO of the above options could be used in a patient with known schizophrenia who requires rapid tranquillisation?

Question 2
Pick one or more options from the following list for each of the questions below:
a) Alcohol
b) Buprenorphine
c) Methadone
d) Naltrexone
e) Cocaine
f) Heroin
g) Diazepam
h) Chlordiazepoxide
i) Disulfiram
j) Korsakoff/Wernicke syndrome
k) Liver cirrhosis
l) Fatty liver
m) Normal liver
n) CAGE
o) TWEAK
p) CAPE

1. A 37-year-old man presents feeling low after the loss of his job. He admits to drinking heavily and that his partner had commented on it. What TWO brief questionnaires could be used to assess whether this patient may have alcohol dependence?
2. A patient with known alcohol dependence syndrome has developed abdominal pain, loss of appetite, fatigue, thirst and light-headedness. He has had an ultrasound scan, and has come to the surgery for his results. What are the most likely results?
3. A 32-year-old patient with a known history of heroin addiction is discussed in clinic, and is eligible for detoxification. He also has a known history of cocaine abuse.
   Which one agent would be most suitable for this purpose?

Question 3

Select one or more options from the list in answer to the following questions:
a) Early morning wakening
b) Feelings of worthlessness
c) Increased energy
d) Increased appetite
e) Decreased sleep
f) Euphoric mood
g) Contact on call psychiatry services for urgent review
h) Refer to outreach team
i) Allow home with advice to return if necessary
j) Fluoxetine
k) Lofepramine
l) Mirtazapine
m) Dosulepin
n) Venlafaxine
o) ECT
p) Diazepam

1. A 28-year-old female patient presents with low mood, anhedonia and negative thoughts toward herself. What THREE other symptoms would you typically expect her to present with?
2. A 46-year-old man, recently divorced, presents with symptoms of depression accompanied by thoughts of self-harm. On closer questioning he has active suicidal ideas and has in fact actioned a plan for suicide by collecting his ex-wife's antidepressant tablets and hoarding them.
   What would be the best course of action in this scenario?
3. A 34-year-old woman presents with low mood and symptoms of moderate to severe depression. She is not actively suicidal and you agree a management plan of drug therapy and talking therapy with her. She has had significant sleep disturbance and would like to have this addressed. What single agent would you try first?

Answers

Single best answer questions

Q1 c.
CBT is a highly effective treatment for anxiety and related disorders as it focuses on the patient's cognitive processes as well as the behavioural responses to these, and how they can be altered.

Q2 a.
Patients who have a BMI < 17.5 are classified as anorexic alongside other diagnostic features.

Q3 d.
Patients in the manic phase of this condition generally sleep less; they may also exhibit flight of ideas, confusion, as well as some psychotic symptoms such as delusions and hallucinations.

Q4 d.
Hypothyroidism is a cause of mental retardation in the antenatal period. Hypoxic insult during the perinatal phase and infections or injury in the postnatal period could also result in mental retardation.

Q5 c.
Psychomotor retardation is a feature of adult depression and not in younger patients. Children may also exhibit poor school performance, school refusal and eating problems.

Q6 c.
Many of the personality disorders (PDs) overlap in some of their features. However, this case clearly describes the main features of a narcissistic personality disorder. The diagnosis of a PD can only be made in the wider context of personality disorder criteria and if shown to be present from early adolescence and even childhood.

Q7 b, c.
The patient is presenting with a condition with a clear onset, there is also a treatable cause for her delirium.

She would not need sedation as she is not showing any disruptive behaviour. In this instance, adequate nursing care and treatment of her infection should suffice in the first instance. Following this she should be re-evaluated.

Q8 b.
This patient most likely has pain in her face secondary to parotid gland enlargement, and the calluses on the backs of her hands are secondary to trauma from the incisors following self-induced vomiting.

Q9 c.

This patient is suffering from a delusion of thought insertion and is also suffering from auditory hallucinations.

Q10 b.

Patients with phobic disorders can be treated with this method which involves patients being gradually exposed to the phobic stimulus to a stage at which they are comfortable; the exposure is increased until the phobia is resolved. Patients only increase their exposure when they are comfortable at each stage.

Q11 d.

Patients with autism are in fact often very distressed by minor changes to their routines.

Q12 a, e.

After initial detention for assessment, patients and healthcare professionals engage in a Mental Health Tribunal to assess for further compulsory detention. The Tribunal is attended by the patient, their representatives, healthcare professionals and independent experts.

Q13 e.

Many psychiatric conditions have been found to have a genetic predisposition, however these findings are yet to yield a clear therapeutic benefit.

Q14 c.

The classic features of school refusal include emotional overprotection, by neurotic parents from a high social class, and schoolwork is usually of a high standard. Truancy is not a feature of typical school refusal.

Q15 d.

Attention deficit hyperactivity disorder is more frequent in learning disabled children, and after prenatal cannabis exposure. Although many parents may suspect behaviour as ADHD, the diagnosis is usually not made until attendance to school, and there is no diagnostic test. There is a familial component, and those affected have a higher risk of suicide and self-harm.

Q16 c.

Night terrors are a common sleep problem among children affecting about 15% of children at some time, usually at age 2–6 years, although can occur at any age. They last less than half an hour and the child usually wakes up screaming and is inconsolable. No treatment is usually required, though rarely sleep medication is used if episodes are very frequent.

Extended matching questions
Question 1
Q1 b, d, h.
In accordance with the ICD 10 criteria, if one of the first four symptoms of thought disorder, delusions of control, auditory hallucinations or other persistent inappropriate delusional ideas are present, then a diagnosis of schizophrenia can be made.

Q2 a, f.
Hypnagogic and hypnopompic hallucinations are present on falling asleep and on waking. These are not considered to be pathological. Secondary delusions are thoughts that develop following an event or experience that results in those thought processes, hence they are not considered as true symptoms of psychiatric disease.

Q3 i, k.
Medical treatment should only be used once other measures have failed; following this, oral therapy should be tried first, and a combination of an antipsychotic and lorazepam often works well. There are, however, more specific regimes for patients with complicated histories including drug abuse, existing combination therapy or severe side effects.

Question 2
Q1 n, o.
The 'CAGE' questionnaire asks about Cutting down, Anger when people comment on alcohol intake, Guilt about drinking and the use of Eye openers in the morning.

'TWEAK' asks about Tolerance, Worry over drinking, Eye openers, Amnesia after drinking and wanting to Cut down.

These methods are useful in the GP consultation, as they can also be recorded for future reference.

Q2 k.
Liver disease becomes symptomatic when permanent damage has developed and the liver is unable to perform its normal functions effectually. This results in the features described above as well as jaundice, ascites and encephalopathy as disease becomes more advanced.

Q3 b.
Methadone can also be used for heroin withdrawal; however, this can be more dangerous in patients who simultaneously use cocaine. In these patients buprenorphine can provide a safer alternative.

Question 3
Q1 a, b, e.
Some patients can develop increased appetite, though it is more common to have reduced appetite and weight loss as a result. In bipolar mood

disorder, euphoria and increased energy can accompany more manic phases in the illness.

Q2 g.
This patient has had a recent life event, and is actively suicidal; more importantly, he has made plans and is acting on them. This patient would be a higher risk of suicide and would need a more detailed assessment from secondary care for the possibility of admission.

Q3 l.
This patient could be tried on mirtazapine as it is effective in those patients with sleep disturbance. Other SSRIs have been shown to cause more sleep disturbance in the initial period of treatment. Many patients may try more than one agent before they settle on one treatment that is effective.

15 Renal Medicine

Single best answer questions

For each question below, what is the most likely answer?
Select ONE option only from the answers supplied.

1. A 35-year-old man presents to the Emergency Department.
   He complains of gradual-onset ankle swelling. On examination
   you note evidence of swelling around his eyes. A urine dipstick
   test demonstrates 3+ protein. What is the most likely diagnosis?
   a) Fraley's syndrome
   b) Goodpasture's syndrome
   c) Glomerulonephritis
   d) Alport's syndrome
   e) Nephrotic syndrome

2. A 42-year-old man presents to the Emergency Department. He
   comments that for the past one week he has been suffering from
   increasing shortness of breath with episodes of coughing up bright
   red blood. He also noticed occasions where he has passed blood
   in his urine. A chest X-ray demonstrates evidence of bilateral patchy
   consolidation. What is the most likely diagnosis?
   a) Alport's syndrome
   b) Balkan nephropathy
   c) Renal cancer
   d) Goodpasture's syndrome
   e) Fraley's syndrome

3. An 8-year-old boy is reviewed in the outpatient department. His mother
   comments that her son no longer seems to respond to his name and
   appears disinterested when asked to do something. On examination you
   note evidence of ankle swelling. A urine dipstick demonstrates evidence
   of 3+ protein and a trace of blood. Fundoscopy reveals fleck-like lesions
   in both retinas. What is the most likely diagnosis?

The Complete GPVTS Stage 2 Preparation Guide: Questions and Professional Dilemmas,
First Edition. Edited by Saba Khan with Neel Sharma.
© 2012 John Wiley & Sons, Ltd. Published 2012 by John Wiley & Sons, Ltd.

a) Alport's syndrome
b) Glomerulonephritis
c) Balkan nephropathy
d) Fraley's syndrome
e) Hyperuricaemic nephropathy

4. A 29-year-old Arabic woman presents to the Emergency Department. She has been suffering from a chest infection for the past few weeks and a fever on and off. She denies any shortness of breath or cough. She informs you that she has noticed episodes of frank blood in her urine which initially resolved but has now returned. She denies any recent travel and is currently not sexually active. What is the most likely diagnosis?
a) Urinary tract infection
b) IgA nephropathy
c) Pneumonia
d) Pyelonephritis
e) Glomerulonephritis

5. A 23-year-old man presents to the Emergency Department. He has been suffering from general fatigue and a sore throat for the past few weeks. Recently he has noticed the presence of blood in his urine. He denies any dysuria or abdominal pain. On examination you note both his eyes are swollen. What is the most likely diagnosis?
a) Post-streptococcal glomerulonephritis
b) Urinary Tract Infection
c) Nephrotic syndrome
d) Pyelonephritis
e) IgA nephropathy

6. A 78-year-old man presents to the Emergency Department. He complains of difficulties in passing urine as well as haematuria. He mentions that he has lost weight recently and has gone off his food. Blood investigations demonstrate a sodium of 143 mmol/L, a potassium of 5.3 mmol/L, a urea of 22 mmol/L and a creatinine of 210 μmol/L. What is the most likely diagnosis?
a) Prostatitis
b) Prostate cancer
c) Benign prostatic hypertrophy
d) Urethritis
e) Glomerulonephritis

7. You are a senior house officer in the renal outpatient setting when your registrar asks you to see the next patient. You are told she is a follow-up patient who suffers from an autosomal recessive disorder, electrolyte abnormalities and muscle weakness. What is the most likely diagnosis?
a) Alport's syndrome
b) Bartter's syndrome

  c) Nephrotic syndrome
  d) Gitelman's syndrome
  e) Fraley's syndrome

8. You are on a post-take ward round when the consultant asks you
   for a diagnosis of a patient he has just seen. He tells you the patient
   suffers from high blood pressure and a low potassium. He continues
   by saying that the patient's serum renin and aldosterone levels
   are both suppressed. What is the most likely diagnosis?
   a) Liddle's syndrome
   b) Bartter's syndrome
   c) Fabry's disease
   d) Fraley's syndrome
   e) Fanconi's syndrome

9. You are on a ward round when your consultant asks you for a
   diagnosis of a patient he has seen. He tells you that the patient
   experiences hypokalaemia due to defective chloride reabsorption
   in the loop of Henle. He continues by saying the patient experiences
   low blood pressure on occasion and has an elevated serum renin
   level. What is the most likely diagnosis?
   a) Fanconi's syndrome
   b) Gitelman's syndrome
   c) Bartter's syndrome
   d) Fraley's syndrome
   e) Liddle's syndrome

10. A 5-year-old boy is reviewed in the Emergency Department. On
    examination you note evidence of abdominal distension and a
    palpable mass in the right flank. He is in a lot of discomfort and
    begins to cry. His mother mentions that she has noticed blood
    in his urine recently. What is the most likely diagnosis?
    a) Renal cyst
    b) Polycystic kidney disease
    c) Hydronephrosis
    d) Wilms' tumour
    e) Crohn disease

11. A 56-year-old man presents to the Emergency Department. He has
    been experiencing nose bleeds for the past few days and episodes
    of haematuria. On examination you note evidence of a saddlenose
    deformity. He has no past medical history and is on no current
    medication. Cardiovascular, respiratory and abdominal examinations
    prove unremarkable. What is the most likely diagnosis?
    a) Wegener's granulomatosis
    b) Acute tubular necrosis
    c) Tuberous sclerosis

d) Goodpasture's syndrome

e) Systemic lupus erythematosus

12. A 20-year-old man presents to the Emergency Department. He complains of fever and weight loss with generalised muscle aches. On examination you note evidence of an urticarial-type rash. Past medical history includes asthma which was diagnosed at birth. Routine blood investigations demonstrate an elevated eosinophil count, with a urea of 15 mmol/L and a creatinine of 242 μmol/L. What is the most likely diagnosis?

a) Systemic lupus erythematosus

b) Churg–Strauss syndrome

c) Prune belly syndrome

d) Acute tubular necrosis

e) IgA nephropathy

13. A 16-year-old boy is seen by his GP. His mother informs the GP that her son has been experiencing episodes of seizures over the past one month. There is no history of epilepsy in the family and he is on no current medication. On examination you note evidence of white patches on his skin. During the consultation the boy mentions he has also been passing frank blood in his urine. He is currently not sexually active. What is the most likely diagnosis?

a) Alport's syndrome

b) Systemic lupus erythematosus

c) Tuberous sclerosis

d) Nephrotic syndrome

e) Acute tubular necrosis

14. A 61-year-old woman with acute on chronic renal failure is reviewed on the post-take ward round. She complains of feeling tired and occasional palpitations. Blood investigations demonstrate a urea of 15 mmol/L, a creatinine of 212 μmol/L, a sodium of 150 mmol/L and a potassium of 7 mmol/L. Which of the following is the most suitable initial management?

a) Calcium gluconate

b) Salbutamol nebulisers

c) Intravenous furosemide 40 mg

d) Insulin and dextrose

e) Calcium resonium, insulin and dextrose

15. A 66-year-old woman is admitted on to the acute medical take with confusion. She has no significant past medical history. Her carer informs you that she has been passing offensive-smelling urine over the past few days. A urine dipstick reveals 3+ leucocytes, 3+ nitrites and 2+ blood. On examination she has a temperature of 40°C, pulse rate of 110 beats per minute and blood pressure of 95/45 mmHg.

She is catheterised and fluid resuscitated. She is commenced on antibiotics intravenously for urosepsis. The next day, routine blood investigations demonstrate a urea of 20 mmol/L and a creatinine of 210 μmol/L. On the day of her admission, blood tests demonstrated normal renal function. What antibiotic is the most likely cause in this case?

a) Penicillin
b) Clarithromycin
c) Vancomycin
d) Gentamicin
e) Metronidazole

Extended matching questions

Question 1
a) Membranous
b) Mesangioproliferative
c) Diffuse proliferative
d) Minimal change disease
e) Focal segmental glomerulosclerosis
f) Rapidly progressive
g) Mesangiocapillary type I
h) Mesangiocapillary type II
i) Mesangiocapillary type V

For each patient below, what is the most likely diagnosis?
Select ONE option only from the list above.
Each option may be selected once, more than once or not at all.

1. A 4-year-old child presenting with hypoalbuminaemia and proteinuria.
2. A patient with a form of glomerulonephritis seen typically in those with hepatitis C infection.
3. A 27-year-old woman presenting with non-specific joint paints, a facial rash and deranged renal function.
4. A 22-year-old man presenting with new-onset haematuria following a recent upper respiratory chest infection.
5. A 65-year-old woman presents to her GP. She complains of generalised swelling and fatigue. A urine dipstick reveals 3+ protein. Past medical history includes rheumatoid arthritis, for which she takes penicillamine.

Question 2
a) Chromosome 16
b) Chromosome 4
c) X-linked recessive
d) X-linked dominant
e) Chromosome 7
f) Autosomal dominant
g) Chromosome 14
h) Autosomal recessive
i) Chromosome 11

For each patient below, what is the most likely genetic association?
Select ONE option only from the list above.
Each option may be selected once, more than once or not at all.

1. A patient with autosomal polycystic kidney disease (APKD) type II.
2. A 23-year-old male presenting with sensorineural deafness and impaired renal function.
3. A young male presenting with new-onset seizures. On examination you note evidence of roughened patches of skin over his lumbar spine.

4. A 6-year-old boy presenting with painless haematuria and an abdominal mass.

5. A patient with a recent diagnosis of liver fibrosis and polcystic kidney disease.

Question 3

a) Wegener's granulomatosis
b) Goodpasture's syndrome
c) Type II renal tubular acidosis
d) Renal calculi
e) Rhabdomyolysis
f) Calcium renal stone disease
g) Type I renal tubular acidosis
h) Urate renal stone disease
i) Type IV renal tubular acidosis

For each patient below, what is the most likely diagnosis?
Select ONE option only from the list above.
Each option may be selected once, more than once or not at all.

1. A 43-year-old man presenting with nasal crusting and epistaxis. On examination you note evidence of a saddle-shaped nose deformity.

2. A 78-year-old woman is admitted to the Emergency Department. You note evidence of impaired renal function but are unable to ascertain a cause currently. She informs you that she has recently been started on a tablet to help lower her cholesterol.

3. A middle-aged man presents with impaired renal function. An arterial blood gas demonstrates a pH of 7.2, a bicarbonate of 18 mmol/L and a base excess of −8 mmol/L. He has recently been diagnosed with rheumatoid arthritis.

4. A 24-year-old male presents to the Emergency Department with impaired renal function. During the consultation he informs you that he tends to experience seizures on occasion, which has been put down to a recently diagnosed liver problem. He is a non-drinker and non-smoker. An arterial blood gas demonstrates evidence of a metabolic acidosis.

5. A middle-aged man presents to the Emergency Department with severe right-sided loin pain. He complains of increased urinary frequency and burning on passing urine. Routine observations reveal a temperature of 38°C. He has recently been seen by the rheumatologists as a result of a red hot swollen right toe.

Answers

Single best answer questions

Q1 e.
This is a typical presentation of nephrotic syndrome which is associated with oedema, proteinuria and a low serum albumin (usually less than 25 g/L). Numerous causes exist including glomerular disease, diabetes, systemic lupus erythematosus, rheumatoid arthritis and drugs such as gold, penicillamine, NSAIDs and captopril. Nephrotic syndrome can result in serious complications such as thrombosis, hyperlipidaemia and acute renal failure.

Q2 d.
Goodpasture's syndrome is an autoimmune disorder associated with autoantibodies directed against type 4 collagen in the glomerular and alveolar basement membrane. It presents with shortness of breath, haemoptysis, haematuria and, in severe cases, massive pulmonary haemorrhage. Treatment comprises steroids, cyclophosphamide or plasma exchange.

Q3 a.
Alport's syndrome is associated with a defect in the alpha-5 chain of type 4 collagen. It is associated with variable thickening and splitting of the glomerular basement membrane. Clinical features include deafness, haematuria which is often microscopic, proteinuria and chronic renal failure. Fundoscopy reveals a 'dot and fleck' type of appearance. Nephrotic syndrome is often seen in a third of individuals.

Q4 b.
IgA nephropathy, also known as Berger's disease, affects young adults in the main. It presents with recurrent haematuria and is associated with an upper respiratory tract infection. It is often seen in the Far East and is associated with IgA deposits in the mesangium. A quarter of individuals may develop end-stage renal failure.

Q5 a.
Presenting features include haematuria and periorbital oedema that occur typically two weeks following a streptococcal infection. In terms of management, salt and water should be restricted, with the use of antihypertensives, in view of possible elevations in blood pressure. Steroids are generally not required.

Q6 b.
This is a classic presentation of prostate cancer. Management relies on surgery or radiotherapy if the malignancy is confined to the gland itself. Metastatic disease involves the use of LHRH analogues.

Q7 d.
Gitelman's syndrome is an autosomal recessive disorder which affects the distal convoluted tubule and is associated with a hypokalaemic metabolic alkalosis as well as hypocalciuria and hypomagnesaemia. Blood pressure is often low or normal. Typical features comprise muscular weakness and tetany. Treatment involves magnesium and potassium supplements.

Q8 a.
Liddle's syndrome is an autosomal dominant condition comprising hypertension, hypokalaemia and a metabolic alkalosis. Renin and aldosterone are typically suppressed. The condition is associated with enhanced reabsorption of sodium in the distal nephron. Treatment consists of salt restriction, potassium supplements and the use of amiloride.

Q9 c.
Bartter's syndrome is associated with defective chloride reabsorption in the loop of Henle. It is associated with low potassium as well as excess renin production with hyperaldosteronism. Treatment involves potassium replacement and NSAIDs.

Q10 d.
Wilms' tumour is a common childhood malignancy associated with WT1 and WT2 gene mutations. Clinical features include abdominal pain, a palpable abdominal mass, haematuria and anaemia. Investigations of choice include an abdominal ultrasound or CT scan with treatment being based on chemotherapy, radiotherapy (in advanced disease) and surgery.

Q11 a.
Wegener's granulomatosis is a necrotising granulomatous vasculitis. It is characterised by epistaxis, purulent nasal discharge and destruction of the nasal septum which gives rise to a saddle-shaped deformity. Renal complications are common and include proteinuria, haematuria and renal failure. Additional features include myalgia, pericarditis, uveitis, scleritis and proptosis.

Q12 b.
The features of Churg–Strauss syndrome comprise asthma, eosinophilia and necrotising glomerulonephritis. Associated complications include rashes, digital ischaemia, myocarditis, gastrointestinal bleeding and peripheral neuropathy.

Q13 c.
Tuberous sclerosis is associated with mutation of *TSC1* or *TSC2* genes. It is associated with neurological complications such as seizures and a diminished IQ. Dermatological features include ash-leaf macules

(described above) and shagreen patches which comprise areas of thick leathery skin found commonly on the back. Renal complications often occur and include haematuria secondary to angiomyolipomas.

Q14 e.
Calcium resonium 15 g orally aids excretion of potassium, as does insulin which helps to drive potassium back into the cells. Salbutamol nebulisers are also a worthwhile treatment option but should not be first line. Calcium gluconate is cardioprotective but does NOT aid in potassium excretion. A high potassium level is a medical emergency and a common cause of cardiorespiratory arrest.

Q15 d.
Gentamicin has profound nephrotoxic effects in the elderly. It should be used with caution and often at a low dose, namely 3 mg/kg, if needed. Additional side effects of gentamicin include hearing loss and loss of balance.

Extended matching questions
Question 1
Q1 d.
Minimal change glomerulonephritis is seen in children typically with nephrotic syndrome. Causes include NSAIDs and Hodgkin's disease. Treatment of choice involves the use of steroids.

Q2 g.
Mesangiocapillary glomerulonephritis type I occurs in cryoglobulinaemia and hepatitis C. Type II is seen in partial lipodystrophy.

Q3 c.
This patient is most likely to be suffering from systemic lupus erythematosus, which results in diffuse proliferative glomerulonephritis most commonly.

Q4 b.
Mesangioproliferative glomerulonephritis is also known as IgA nephropathy or Berger's disease. It occurs commonly in young adults and presents with haematuria following a chest infection.

Q5 a.
Membranous glomerulonephritis is commonly seen following the use of rheumatoid drugs and also in malignancy. It typically presents as nephrotic syndrome. The prognosis of the condition is remembered using the 'rule of thirds' approach:

1/3 of cases resolve spontaneously;
1/3 of cases continue to have persistent proteinuria;
1/3 of cases develop end-stage renal failure.

Question 2

Q1 b.

APKD type I is linked to chromosome 16 and type II is associated with gene defects on chromosome 4.

Q2 b.

This patient has Alport's syndrome, an X-linked dominant condition. It presents with microscopic haematuria, renal failure, bilateral sensorineural deafness and retinitis pigmentosa.

Q3 f.

This patient has tuberous sclerosis, an autosomal dominant condition. It presents with seizures, cutaneous abnormalities including café-au-lait patches and polcystic kidneys.

Q4 i.

The most likely diagnosis in this case is a Wilms' tumour. It presents with an abdominal mass, painless haematuria and flank pain. Over one-third of cases are associated with a mutation of the *WT1* gene located on chromosome 11.

Q5 h.

Autosomal recessive polycystic kidney disease is likely in this case. It presents with impaired renal function and liver fibrosis. It is commonly due to a gene defect localised to chromosome 6.

Question 3

Q1 a.

Wegener's granulomatosis presents with epistaxis, sinusitis and glomerulonephritis. Investigations demonstrate a positive cANCA and chest X-ray is likely to demonstrate evidence of cavitation. Treatment relies on the use of steroids or plasma exchange.

Q2 e.

This patient is likely to have rhabdomyolysis secondary to her recent use of a statin. Patients present with impaired renal function, elevated creatine kinase and low calcium. Intravenous fluid replacement is the treatment of choice.

Q3 g.

Type I renal tubular acidosis is commonly seen in those with rheumatoid arthritis, systemic lupus erythematosus and Sjogren's syndrome. Complications include renal stone formation.

Q4 c.

Type II renal tubular acidosis is seen commonly in Wilson's disease which is the likely diagnosis in the above patient. It is associated with reduced reabsorption of bicarbonate in the proximal tubule and a low serum potassium.

Q5 h.

This man is likely to be suffering from gout in view of his swollen right toe. Gout is a risk factor for the formation of urate stones. Treatment of choice includes allopurinol and oral bicarbonate.

16 Reproductive Health

For each question below, what is the most likely answer?
Select ONE option only from the answers supplied.

1. You are an F2 doctor working in general practice. A woman attends for
   a 6-week postnatal check. She requests contraception. What would you
   recommend?
   a) The combined oral contraceptive pill
   b) The progesterone-only pill
   c) No contraception is needed as she is postpartum and is protected

2. Which is the most common cause of amenorrhoea?
   a) Pregnancy
   b) Anorexia nervosa
   c) Polycystic ovarian syndrome
   d) Endometriosis

3. What is oligomenorrhoea?
   a) Painful periods
   b) Heavy periods
   c) Irregular periods

4. Which of the following can present as postcoital bleeding?
   a) *Chlamydia* infection
   b) Polyps
   c) Cervical cancer
   d) All of the above

5. You are working in general practice. A 35-year-old married woman
   attends with a 3-month history of spotting in between her periods. She
   is using barrier contraception and a home pregnancy test was negative.
   You perform a bimanual and speculum examination, which are normal.
   What is your management plan?

The Complete GPVTS Stage 2 Preparation Guide: Questions and Professional Dilemmas,
First Edition. Edited by Saba Khan with Neel Sharma.
© 2012 John Wiley & Sons, Ltd. Published 2012 by John Wiley & Sons, Ltd.

a) Refer for colposcopy
b) Perform a smear test and take swabs
c) Send her for some blood tests
d) Arrange an ultrasound scan

6. You are working in general practice. You see a 26-year-old girl who requests the 'morning-after' pill. She last had unprotected sexual intercourse 48 hours ago, and her last menstrual period was 2 weeks ago. It is the third time she has used emergency contraception. What is your course of action?
   a) You refuse to issue it as she has had it already
   b) You prescribe Levonelle (levonorgestrel 1.5 mg single dose)
   c) You offer her Levonelle or the intrauterine device
   d) You suggest she start taking the combined oral contraceptive pill

7. You are an F2 doctor working in general practice. You see a 28-year-old man with a history of urethral discharge and mild dysuria. He has no other urinary symptoms. He is sexually active. What is the most useful investigation?
   a) Urethral swab
   b) Urinalysis
   c) Penile swab
   d) Rectal swab

8. You are an F2 doctor working in the maternity day unit. A patient with a headache and visual symptoms is referred by her GP. She is a 32-week primigravida. What two first-line bedside tests should you carry out?
   a) Temperature and urine dipstick test for proteinuria
   b) Blood pressure and oxygen saturation
   c) Heart rate and blood pressure
   d) Blood pressure and urine dipstick test for proteinuria
   e) Urine dipstick for glucosuria and blood pressure

9. You are an F2 doctor working in general practice. You see a 30-year-old woman who is 8 weeks pregnant. She has experienced some vaginal bleeding and lower abdominal pain which is also felt in her shoulder tip. Her blood pressure is 100/60 mmHg and her pulse rate is 110 beats per minute. What is your differential diagnosis and management?
   a) Ectopic pregnancy: refer to the early pregnancy unit
   b) Threatened miscarriage: refer to the early pregnancy unit
   c) Ovarian cyst: arrange admission to hospital
   d) Ectopic pregnancy: refer to the gynaecology team and arrange urgent admission
   e) Appendicitis: refer to the surgical team and arrange urgent admission

10. What are the contraindications to hormone replacement therapy?
    a) Age < 45 years
    b) An undiagnosed breast mass
    c) A family history of fibroids
    d) Gilbert syndrome

11. You are an F2 working in general practice. You see a 60-year-old woman with a 2-month history of abdominal bloating, general malaise and weight loss. She has also noticed a small amount of dark brown discharge. On examination you feel a pelvic mass. What first-line investigation(s) should be done?
    a) Abdominal X-ray
    b) Ca125 and ultrasound scan
    c) Smear test
    d) MRI scan
    e) Colposcopy

12. You are an F2 doctor working in general practice. You see a 25-year-old with a long history of menorrhagia. Her periods are regular and she has never been sexually active. She has no other past medical history. Recent blood tests and a pelvic ultrasound were normal. She is not keen on hormonal treatment. What would you prescribe for her heavy periods?
    a) Microgynon
    b) Mefenamic acid
    c) Mirena intrauterine system

13. Which of the following forms part of routine antenatal screening?
    a) Full blood count and blood group
    b) HIV status
    c) Rubella status
    d) Syphilis status
    e) All of the above

14. You are an F2 doctor working in the Emergency Department. A 28-year-old woman who is 35/40 comes in with an episode of vaginal bleeding. She has been told she has a low-lying placenta. She is haemodynamically stable and the bleeding has stopped. What is your management?
    a) The bleeding has resolved so she can be discharged with antenatal follow-up
    b) Establish intravenous access and admit her to the obstetric ward
    c) Organise an ultrasound scan at 36 weeks to check placental position
    d) Check her haemoglobin and discharge her if it is normal

15. Which of the following are fetal complications of maternal diabetes?
    a) Congenital abnormalities
    b) Low birth weight
    c) Oligohydramnios
    d) Hypothyroidism

Extended matching questions

Question 1
What is the most likely cause of pelvic pain in the following scenarios?
Choose from the list below.
a) Pelvic inflammatory disease
b) Ovarian cyst accident
c) Ectopic pregnancy
d) Carcinoma
e) Polycystic ovarian syndrome
f) Uterine fibroids
g) Endometriosis
h) Miscarriage
i) Irritable bowel syndrome
j) Adenomyosis
k) Inflammatory bowel disease
l) Appendicitis
m) Endometrial polyp

1. Your patient is a 26-year-old woman with painful periods and deep dyspareunia. The pain often starts before the onset of menstruation and she has noticed spotting in between her periods. A recent sexual health screen was normal. Which option is the most likely diagnosis?
2. Your patient is a 22-year-old woman with a 3-day history of bilateral lower abdominal pain, discharge and deep dyspareunia. Her last menstrual period was 5 days ago and she has recently changed sexual partners. She is not currently using any contraception. What is the most likely diagnosis?
3. Your patient is a 33-year-old woman with a 24-hour history of acute right iliac fossa pain. It started suddenly and is very severe. She has had an appendicectomy in the past. Her urinary BHCG is negative. What is the most probable diagnosis?

Question 2
What is the most likely cause of vaginal discharge in the following scenarios? Choose from the list below.
a) Carcinoma
b) Physiological
c) Bacterial vaginosis
d) Fistula
e) Gonorrhea
f) Oral contraceptive pill
g) *Trichomonas vaginalis*
h) Chemical vaginitis
i) *Candida albicans*
j) Foreign body
k) Cervical polyp
l) Intrauterine device
m) *Chlamydia*

1. A 29-year-old woman attends the surgery with a 4-day history of an offensive green discharge and superficial dyspareunia. A speculum reveals a punctate erythematous cervix with a strawberry appearance. What is the most likely cause?
2. A 35-year-old woman who is 20/40 has noticed an itchy white vaginal discharge. It is not foul-smelling. She has recently completed a course of antibiotics for a chest infection. What is the most likely diagnosis?
3. A 25-year-old woman notices a fishy grey discharge. It is not itchy or painful. What is the most likely cause of this symptom?

Question 3

What is the most suitable method of contraception in the following scenarios? Choose from the list below.
a) Cervical cap
b) Cerazette
c) Depot injection
d) Vasectomy
e) Progesterone-only pill
f) Emergency contraception
g) Abstinence
h) Mirena intrauterine system
i) Female sterilisation
j) Combined oral contraceptive pill
k) Implanon
l) Copper intrauterine device
m) Oestrogen patch
n) Condoms

1. Your patient is a 32-year-old married woman with a history of migraine with aura. She would like to start planning a family soon but would like a reliable form of contraception in the interim. She is allergic to latex. What is the most suitable option?
2. Your patient is a 20-year-old woman who was previously on the pill but frequently missed her tablets. She is in a stable relationship and is not planning a family. She is otherwise well. She hates having her smear tests as she finds them very uncomfortable. What is the best option for her?
3. Your patient is a 36-year-old woman with a history of menorrhagia due to fibroids. She is in a stable relationship and has completed her family. She is a smoker. She is not keen on surgery. What is the best method for this patient?

Answers

Single best answer questions

Q1 b.
Without further information about whether she is exclusively breastfeeding, answer c) is incorrect. The combined pill is not recommended in the first 6 weeks as it can adversely affect milk volume if breastfeeding and is outside product licence.

Q2 a.
All answers can cause loss of menstruation. Excessive weight loss and intensive exercise commonly cause amenorrhoea in athletes or in women with eating disorders.

Q3 c.
Painful periods are termed dysmenorrhoea while menorrhagia describes excessive blood loss during menstruation.

Q4 d.
Commonly it is caused by cervical trauma or a cervical ectropion.

Q5 b.
Causes for intermenstrual bleeding are similar to those causing postcoital bleeding and include *Chlamydia* infection, cervical polyps, ectropion, cervicitis, vaginitis and cervical cancer. In the first instance, a smear should be performed and a high vaginal and endocervical swab or urine sample sent for polymerase chain reaction (PCR) testing to exclude *Chlamydia*. Colposcopy may be indicated depending on examination findings and the presence of risk factors for carcinoma.

Q6 c.
Emergency contraception is indicated. If it is more than 72 hours after unprotected intercourse, the progesterone-only emergency contraception is not recommended and the patient should be referred for insertion of the copper intrauterine device. In this case, the patient should be offered both. A sexual infection screen should be considered and you should discuss future contraception.

Q7 a.
The presence of a discharge suggests acute urethritis and urethral swabs should include swabs for *Gonococcus* and *Chlamydia*. A first-pass urine examination is also important to exclude a urinary tract infection. A full sexual history should be taken.

Q8 d.
Pre-eclampsia is a multisystem disorder which resolves after delivery. It is one the most important causes of maternal death and screening involves regular antenatal blood pressure readings and urinalysis. Eclampsia

describes a fit as a result of pre-eclampsia. Symptoms of pre-eclampsia include headache, oedema, visual symptoms, abdominal pain and vomiting.

Q9 d.
Ectopic pregnancy should always be suspected if pain is felt in the shoulder tip, fainting episode, tenderness on abdominal or pelvic examination. In this case, the patient is hypotensive and tachycardic so urgent admission is warranted. An ovarian cyst accident and threatened miscarriage can also present with pain and bleeding but in this case an ectopic pregnancy must first be excluded. Appendicitis rarely causes bleeding.

Q10 b.
Absolute contraindications to HRT include current breast or endometrial cancer, severe active liver disease and venous or arterial thrombosis. Gilbert syndrome is an inherited disorder causing an isolated unconjugated hyperbilirubinaemia and requires no treatment.

Q11 b.
This patient should be referred for suspected gynaecological malignancy as a 2-week rule. She has features indicative of ovarian carcinoma.

Q12 b.
This patient has dysfunctional uterine bleeding, a diagnosis of exclusion and a common cause for menorrhagia. All answers are possible treatments for menorrhagia, but patient preference has to be taken into account. A sensible first-line choice would be mefenamic acid 500 mg tds starting on the first day of her period and to be taken on the days of heavy flow. Tranexamic acid is an alternative. Microgynon is a combined oral contraceptive pill and can be used for cycle control.

Q13 e.
Other basic screening tests include hepatitis B status, antibody status, urinalysis.

Q14 b.
This woman has had an antepartum haemorrhage with a possible placenta praevia. A full blood count, clotting and cross-match are needed; fetal wellbeing is assessed with cardiotocography (CTG). An ultrasound will determine the exact position of the placenta. Placenta praevia is classified according to the proximity of the placenta to the internal os of the cervix. If she is rhesus-negative, anti-D is administered. The patient is at risk of massive haemorrhage and needs to be admitted for observation. Delivery is by elective caesarean section.

Q15 a.
Macrosomia, polyhydramnios and preterm labour are common complications. Birth trauma, especially shoulder dystocia, is more common in these babies.

Extended matching questions
Question 1
Q1 g.
Endometriosis is the presence of endometrial tissue outside the uterus.
It is often asymptomatic. When present, symptoms include dysmenorrhoea,
dyspareunia, pelvic pain, subfertility and menstrual problems. Diagnosis is
by laparoscopy.

Q2 a.
Pelvic inflammatory disease is an important cause of subfertility.
Chlamydia and gonococcus are usually implicated. When severe, it can
cause high fever, tachycardia, peritonism and endometritis. Treatment is
with antibiotics given intravenously in severe cases.

Q3 b.
Both an ovarian cyst rupture or torsion are differentials although the
former is more common.

Question 2
Q1 g.
This sexually transmitted infection is relatively uncommon in the UK. It is
caused by a flagellate protozoan and is treated with metronidazole.

Q2 i.
Thrush is common. Risk factors include the oral contraceptive pill,
pregnancy, antibiotics and diabetes.

Q3 c.
Bacterial vaginosis occurs when the normal vaginal flora is disrupted
and there is overgrowth of mixed flora including anaerobes
(*Gardnerella* and *Mycoplasma hominis*). It is characterised by a fishy
discharge and 'clue cells' on microscopy. Treatment is with
metronidazole.

Question 3
Q1 e or b.
Due to the history of migraine with aura, the combined pill is
contraindicated. Long-acting reversible methods are unsuitable as this
patient is requesting a short-term option. Given her allergy to latex and
need for a reliable method, the best option would be the progesterone-
only pill.

Q2 c or k.
A long-acting method would suit this patient as compliance is a problem.
The depot injection is probably the best choice but the implant would also
be a good option. From the scenario, an intrauterine device insertion may
not be tolerated or preferred.

Q3 h.

The Mirena intrauterine system is a good option as it will address her menorrhagia as well as contraceptive needs. She is over 35 and a smoker, therefore the combined pill would not be the safest option. She has completed her family and, although further discussion is needed, vasectomy would be an option that she could discuss with her partner.

17 Respiratory Medicine

For each question below, what is the most likely answer?
Select ONE option only from the answers supplied.

1. A 69-year-old man is referred to the Emergency Department by his GP. He complains of gradual-onset shortness of breath and a cough productive of yellow sputum. On examination you note reduced breath sounds over the right base. A chest X-ray confirms evidence of a right-sided pleural effusion. You perform a diagnostic tap and aspirate 100 mL of straw-coloured fluid. The pH of the aspirate is noted to be 7.2. What is the most likely diagnosis?
   a) Lung cancer
   b) Pleural empyema
   c) Haemothorax
   d) Chylothorax
   e) Pneumothorax

2. A 79-year-old man is admitted to hospital. He complains of worsening shortness of breath and chest pain. On examination you note he is cachectic and has evidence of reduced air entry on the left base. A chest X-ray shows evidence of a left-sided pleural effusion and bilateral pleural thickening. What is the most likely diagnosis?
   a) Asthma
   b) Mesothelioma
   c) Chronic obstructive pulmonary disease
   d) Pneumonia
   e) Tuberculosis

3. A 75-year-old woman presents to the GP. She complains of shortness of breath and a productive cough. She has been a long-term smoker and still continues to smoke. Chest examination demonstrates evidence of hyperexpansion with no tracheal deviation. What is the most likely diagnosis?

The Complete GPVTS Stage 2 Preparation Guide: Questions and Professional Dilemmas,
First Edition. Edited by Saba Khan with Neel Sharma.
© 2012 John Wiley & Sons, Ltd. Published 2012 by John Wiley & Sons, Ltd.

a) Asthma
b) Pneumonia
c) Empyema
d) Chronic obstructive pulmonary disease
e) Lung cancer

4. A 56-year-old woman presents to her GP. She complains of gradual-onset chest pain over the past two weeks. On examination she is tender over her chest wall with evidence of a discrete swelling in the region of the second and third ribs. She has recently undergone radiotherapy for breast cancer. What is the most likely diagnosis?
   a) Pulmonary embolism
   b) Pneumothorax
   c) Tietze syndrome
   d) Sarcoidosis
   e) Pneumonia

5. A 62-year-old man presents to the Emergency Department. He has been suffering from a productive cough of rusty-brown-coloured sputum and a fever for the past 1 week. He is a long-term injecting drug abuser. He denies any episodes of night sweats or weight loss. On examination you note a temperature of 39°C. What is the most likely diagnosis?
   a) Tuberculosis
   b) *Staphylococcus* pneumonia
   c) Lung cancer
   d) *Legionella* pneumonia
   e) Chronic obstructive pulmonary disease

6. A 45-year-old woman is admitted to the Emergency Department with increasing shortness of breath. On examination her oxygen saturations are 89% on room air with a respiratory rate of 29 breaths per minute and pulse rate of 112 beats per minute. Chest auscultation reveals the presence of an inspiratory wheeze bilaterally. An arterial blood gas demonstrates a pO_2 of 8.9 kPa. She is a long-term smoker but informs you that she has recently stopped smoking 1 week ago. What is the most likely diagnosis?
   a) Pneumonia
   b) Pneumothorax
   c) Sarcoidosis
   d) Asthma
   e) Pulmonary embolism

7. A 76-year-old woman is seen by her GP. She complains of gradual-onset pain in her left shoulder which spreads to her ring fingers. She is a long-term smoker since her early teens and still continues to smoke. On examination you note evidence of drooping of the upper eyelid on the left side. What is the most likely diagnosis?

a) Sarcoidosis
b) Asbestosis
c) Horner's syndrome
d) Tuberculosis
e) Pancoast tumour

8. A 16-year-old boy attends the Emergency Department having been stabbed in the right side of his chest while walking home late at night. On examination he is severely short of breath. General observations reveal a respiratory rate of 29 breaths per minute and oxygen saturations of 89% on room air. Examination of his chest reveals dullness to percussion on the right side with decreased breath sounds. What is the most likely diagnosis?
a) Pneumothorax
b) Haemothorax
c) Flail chest
d) Chylothorax
e) Pulmonary embolism

9. You are the F2 doctor on call when a nurse asks you to see a patient with sudden-onset shortness of breath. Reading her admission notes you note that she was originally admitted with right leg swelling and cellulitis, for which she is on intravenous antibiotics. Past medical history reveals a fractured right neck of femur which was treated surgically 4 weeks prior. On examination you note a respiratory rate of 28 breaths per minute and oxygen saturations of 89% on room air. Chest auscultation is clear with no crepitations or wheeze. What is the most likely diagnosis?
a) Pneumothorax
b) Deep vein thrombosis
c) Pulmonary embolism
d) Pneumonia
e) Asthma

10. A 32-year-old man attends the Emergency Department with a 2-week history of shortness of breath and a non-productive cough. He has recently been on holiday to Dubai and states that he spent most of his time indoors as it was very humid. On chest examination you note evidence of crepitations on his left base. What is the most likely diagnosis?
a) Tuberculosis
b) Pulmonary fibrosis
c) Sarcoidosis
d) *Staphylococcus* pneumonia
e) *Legionella* pneumonia

11. A 75-year-old man is admitted to the Emergency Department with shortness of breath. He has a background history of congestive cardiac

failure. A chest X-ray demonstrates evidence of significant bibasal pleural effusions. A pleural tap is performed and a repeat chest X-ray ordered. Two hours later the patient complains of severe chest pain and increasing shortness of breath. Oxygen saturations are 87% on room air. What is the most likely diagnosis?
a) Intractable heart failure
b) Pulmonary embolism
c) Pneumonia
d) Pneumothorax
e) Myocardial infarction

12. A 73-year-old long-term smoker presents to the Emergency Department with increasing shortness of breath and haemoptysis. On examination you note he is severely cachectic and has finger clubbing. Chest auscultation is unremarkable. During your assessment he states that he has also been finding it difficult to pass motion but denies any abdominal pain. What is the most likely diagnosis?
a) Chronic obstructive pulmonary disease
b) Goodpasture's syndrome
c) Pulmonary embolism
d) Lung cancer
e) Tuberculosis

13. A 52-year-year-old man presents with shortness of breath and frothy sputum. On examination you note crepitations bibasally and minimal ankle oedema. Oxygen saturations are 91% on room air with a respiratory rate of 28 breaths per minute. What is the most likely explanation for the patient's symptoms?
a) Pulmonary embolism
b) Tuberculosis
c) Asthma
d) Pulmonary oedema
e) Chronic obstructive pulmonary disease

14. A 42-year-old man presents to the respiratory outpatient department complaining of shortness of breath and generalised joint pains. On examination you note evidence of a purple discolouration of his nose and forehead. A recent chest X-ray demonstrates evidence of bilateral hilar lymphadenopathy. What is the most likely diagnosis?
a) Pneumonia
b) Sarcoidosis
c) Asbestosis
d) Costochondritis
e) Goodpasture's syndrome

15. A 72-year-old man presents to the Emergency Department with worsening shortness of breath. He is known to suffer from inflammatory bowel disease, for which he takes methotrexate.

On chest examination you note evidence of bibasal inspiratory crackles. What is the most likely diagnosis?
a) Pneumonia
b) Pulmonary fibrosis
c) Pneumothorax
d) Goodpasture's syndrome
e) Wegener's syndrome

Extended matching questions

Question 1
a) Asbestosis
b) Berylliosis
c) Mesothelioma
d) Silicosis
e) Pneumonia
f) Sarcoidosis
g) Chronic obstructive pulmonary disease
h) Coal workers' pneumoconiosis
i) Emphysema

For each patient below, what is the most likely diagnosis?
Select ONE option only from the list above.
Each option may be selected once, more than once or not at all.

1. A 72-year-old retired coal miner presents with shortness of breath and a dry cough. A chest X-ray demonstrates evidence of small round opacities in both lung fields.
2. A 75-year-old retired sandblaster is admitted with increasing shortness of breath and a dry cough. A chest X-ray demonstrates evidence of nodules in the upper lobes.
3. A 78-year-old retired shipyard worker presents with increasing shortness of breath. On examination you note evidence of lower zone crepitations on chest auscultation. A chest X-ray reveals a honeycomb pattern. He denies any weight loss.
4. A 47-year-old man presents to the Emergency Department. He complains of shortness of breath in addition to a cough and generalised joint pains. He works as a ceramic manufacturer. On examination you note evidence of inspiratory crackles. A chest X-ray demonstrates evidence of bilateral hilar lymphadenopathy.
5. A 35-year-old Afro-Caribbean woman presents to the Emergency Department. She complains of a dry cough and shortness of breath. She denies any weight loss. On examination you note evidence of finger clubbing and erythematous lesions on her lower limbs.

Question 2
a) *Chlamydia* pneumonia
b) Chronic obstructive pulmonary disease
c) *Mycoplasma* pneumonia
d) *Legionella* pneumonia
e) Cystic fibrosis
f) *Pneumocystis jiroveci* pneumonia
g) Empyema
h) *Staphylococcus aureus* pneumonia
i) Pneumonia

For each patient below, what is the most likely diagnosis?
Select ONE option only from the list above.
Each option may be selected once, more than once or not at all.

1. A 19-year-old female presents to the Emergency Department. She complains of a cough productive of sputum. On examination you note evidence of erythematous lesions on her lower limbs. Blood investigations demonstrate the presence of cold agglutinins.
2. A 45-year-old man presents to the Emergency Department complaining of a cough productive of green sputum. He has recently been abroad to Egypt and comments that he spent most of his time enjoying the hotel's leisure facilities. Blood investigations demonstrate a serum sodium of 129 mmol/L.
3. A 43-year-old Afro-Caribbean man is admitted to the Emergency Department. He is severely short of breath. On examination you note oxygen saturations of 94% on room air which decrease on mobilisation. He comments that he has been unfaithful to his wife on more than one occasion.
4. A 31-year-old injecting drug abuser presents with a cough productive of foul-smelling sputum. On examination you note evidence of right basal crepitations. A chest X-ray confirms evidence of consolidation on the right base.
5. A 47-year-old man presents with shortness of breath and a non-productive cough. During the consultation he states that he has been experiencing neck stiffness for the past two weeks. He is known to be a fond admirer of parrots and has several different species in his flat.

Question 3
a) Pneumothorax
b) Cystic fibrosis
c) Chronic obstructive pulmonary disease
d) Lung cancer
e) Sarcoidosis
f) Tuberculosis
g) Asthma
h) Pleural effusion
i) Pulmonary embolism

For each patient below, what is the most likely diagnosis?
Select ONE option only from the list above.
Each option may be selected once, more than once or not at all.

1. A 25-year-old Nigerian woman presents to the Emergency Department. She complains of a 1-week history of haemoptysis, night sweats and weight loss. She states that at times her night sweats are so severe that her bed sheets are drenched in sweat.

2. A 19-year-old male presents to his GP. He complains of worsening shortness of breath over the past one month. He goes on to mention that he has noticed his stools are offensive in nature and difficult to flush on occasion.

3. A 65-year-old long-term smoker presents with shortness of breath. On examination you note scattered crepitations on chest auscultation bilaterally. Oxygen saturations are 91% on room air. A chest X-ray demonstrates hyperexpanded lung fields.

4. A 34-year-old woman presents to the Emergency Department with sudden-onset shortness of breath. She complains of chest pain on inspiration which she describes as sharp in nature. Current medication includes the oral contraceptive pill. Oxygen saturations are 89% on room air. An arterial blood gas demonstrates a pO_2 of 8 kPa on room air.

5. A 43-year-old man with a background history of cirrhosis presents with shortness of breath. On examination you note decreased breath sounds on the left with dullness to percussion and decreased tactile fremitus.

Answers

Single best answer questions
Q1 b.

A pleural empyema is a collection of pus in the pleural cavity. The fluid is of low pH, low glucose, high lactate dehydrogenase (LDH) and elevated protein. Treatment of choice includes insertion of a chest drain and intravenous antibiotics. Lung cancer is likely to present with shortness of breath, weight loss and haemoptysis. A haemothorax is an accumulation of blood in the thoracic cavity which occurs secondary to trauma, malignancy or tuberculosis. A chylothorax is associated with the presence of lymphatic fluid in the pleural space secondary to leakage from the thoracic duct. Patients present with dyspnoea or tachypnoea. A pneumothorax is associated with shortness of breath and chest pain. Examination findings reveal absent breath sounds, hyper-resonance on chest wall percussion and asymmetrical lung expansion.

Q2 b.

These are classic X-ray findings of mesothelioma, a condition associated with malignant cell transformation within the pleura and seen secondary to asbestos exposure. Clinical features include dyspnoea, chest pain, fever and weight loss. Surgical intervention is typically the mainstay form of treatment. Chronic obstructive pulmonary disease (COPD) presents as hyperexpanded lung fields on a chest X-ray. Pneumonia will demonstrate evidence of consolidation and tuberculosis the presence of cavitating lesions, infiltrates or nodules. A chest X-ray in asthma is often normal but is required to rule out the presence of a pneumothorax.

Q3 d.

COPD is seen in long-term smokers. A chest X-ray will demonstrate hyperexpanded lung fields. Patients presenting with an exacerbation of COPD are managed with steroids, nebulised salbutamol and ipratropium bromide as well as antibiotics if deemed infective.

Q4 c.

Tietze syndrome is associated with inflammation of the costal cartilages. It is differentiated from costochondritis due to the presence of swelling. It can occur following radiotherapy to the chest region as well as after minor injury or strain to the chest wall. Sarcoidosis presents with shortness of breath, fever and joint discomfort. Chest X-ray findings include bilateral hilar lymphadenopathy, infiltrates and fibrosis.

Q5 b.

Staphylococcus pneumonia is often seen in injecting drug abusers. Treatment of choice includes flucloxacillin intravenously. Tuberculosis presents with haemoptysis, night sweats, fever and weight loss. *Legionella* pneumonia can arise from contaminated water sources, for example cooling systems and whirlpool spas. Patients present with headaches, fever and gastrointestinal symptoms such as nausea and diarrhoea. Treatment of choice includes levofloxacin or azithromycin.

Q6 d.

This is a classic presentation of an asthma exacerbation. Treatment of choice would include high-flow oxygen, steroids intravenously, antibiotics and nebulised bronchodilators. In accordance with the British Thoracic Society criteria, a severe attack of asthma comprises:

PEF 33–50% of predicted
Respiratory rate > 25 breaths per minute
Heart rate > 110 beats per minute
Inability to complete sentences in one breath

Life-threatening asthma comprises:

PEF < 33% of predicted
$pO_2 < 8\,kPa$
Normal pCO_2
Silent chest
Cyanosis
Poor respiratory effort
Exhaustion, altered level of consciousness

Q7 e.

A Pancoast tumour comprises a mass within the thoracic inlet and produces symptoms due to involvement of the eighth cranial nerve roots, first and second thoracic trunk and sympathetic chain. Horner's syndrome is a common occurrence secondary to sympathetic chain involvement and comprises miosis, ptosis and anhidrosis.

Q8 b.

Trauma is the number one cause of a haemothorax whereby there is accumulation of blood in the pleural cavity. Flail chest is also seen following chest trauma but results in a paradoxical motion of the affected chest wall segment while breathing.

Q9 c.

Recent surgery in this patient has resulted in a deep vein thrombosis and subsequent pulmonary embolus. The investigation of choice would be a computed tomographic pulmonary angiography (CTPA) and treatment with enoxaparin 1.5 mg/kg.

Q10 e.

Legionella pneumonia is associated with contaminated water sources, for example cooling systems, showers and whirlpool spas. A non-productive cough is a common occurrence. Gastrointestinal symptoms are also common, in particular diarrhoea and vomiting. Antibiotics, namely levofloxacin and azithromycin, are the mainstay form of treatment.

Q11 d.

This patient has developed a pneumothorax following pleural aspiration. A chest drain should be inserted immediately with high-flow oxygen to prevent respiratory arrest.

Q12 d.

The most likely diagnosis here is lung cancer in view of the patient's weight loss and haemoptysis. The patient is also constipated, which is often seen in malignancy, due to an elevated serum calcium. Goodpasture's syndrome comprises pulmonary haemorrhage, glomerulonephritis and anti-GBM antibodies. Treatment of choice includes steroids and cyclophosphamide.

Q13 d.

This is a classic presentation of pulmonary oedema. A chest X-ray is likely to show an enlarged heart, linear pulmonary opacities and pleural effusions. High-flow oxygen is essential in terms of management, as well as intravenous furosemide and, in severe cases, a glyceryl trinitrate (GTN) infusion.

Q14 b.

Sarcoidosis is a multisystem inflammatory disorder which affects the lungs and intrathoracic lymph nodes. Presenting features include a cough, chest pain, fever and arthralgia. Additional features include erythema nodosum, lupus pernio (described above) as well as ocular, neurological and cardiac complications. Bilateral hilar lymphadenopathy is a typical chest X-ray finding. Treatment includes corticosteroids.

Q15 b.

Pulmonary fibrosis tends to present with inspiratory crepitations that sound similar to Velcro. Numerous causes exist including drugs such as methotrexate and amiodarone, as well as genetic factors, smoking and reflux disease. A chest X-ray is likely to demonstrate reticular opacities and honeycombing. Steroids and other immunosuppressive therapies such as azathioprine may prove worthwhile.

Extended matching questions
Question 1
Q1 h.

Coal workers' pneumoconiosis presents typically 10–20 years after coal exposure. It results in small round opacities on the chest X-ray. Spirometry reveals a mixed obstructive and restrictive lung pattern. A complication of the condition is progressive massive fibrosis. Treatment relies on oxygen and bronchodilators.

Q2 d.
Silicosis is seen after inhalation of silicon dioxide in rockface miners, quarry workers and sandblasters. It initially presents with shortness of breath and a dry cough. Pulmonary function testing reveals a restrictive pattern. It is associated with upper lobe nodule formation and the only treatment of choice is lung transplantation.

Q3 a.
Asbestosis is commonly seen 20 years after exposure. It is associated with lower lobe fibrosis. Presenting features include a dry cough, exertional shortness of breath and finger clubbing. A chest X-ray reveals a honeycomb appearance. Pulmonary function tests reveal a restrictive pattern and low carbon monoxide transfer coefficient (KCO).

Q4 b.
Berylliosis is seen commonly in those who work in the electronic, fibreoptic or ceramic industry. It is associated with non-caseating granulomas and fibrous lymph node changes. A chest X-ray will often demonstrate evidence of bilateral hilar lymphadenopathy and fine nodules. Steroids are the mainstay form of treatment.

Q5 f.
Sarcoidosis is a multisystem disease seen commonly in Afro-Caribbean individuals. It is associated with non-caseating granulomas and presents with shortness of breath and a dry cough. A chest X-ray demonstrates evidence of bilateral hilar lymphadenopathy. Additional features include arrhythmias, erythema nodosum, splenomegaly, meningitis and arthritis. Blood investigations demonstrate an elevated serum calcium and serum ACE. Transbronchial biopsy is diagnostic. The management of choice is steroids.

Question 2
Q1 c.
Mycoplasma pneumonia is seen commonly in young adults. Cold agglutinins occur in 50% of cases. Additional features include myocarditis, erythema nodosum, thrombocytopenia and neuropathies.

Q2 d.
Legionella pneumonia is seen following contact with contaminated water cooling systems, showers and air conditioning systems. Additional features include diarrhoea, confusion and headaches. There is often a low serum sodium level secondary to SIADH (syndrome of inappropriate ADH secretion) with thrombocytopenia. *Legionella* antigens may be detected in the urine.

Q3 f.
This picture is commonly seen in individuals with HIV infection.
A drop in oxygen saturations on exercise is typical of the condition.
Diagnosis involves confirmation of the organism in sputum samples or
following bronchoalveolar lavage. Treatment relies upon the use of
cotrimoxazole.

Q4 h.
This form of pneumonia is often seen in injecting drug misusers. A chest
X-ray demonstrates patchy infiltrates with complications such as abscess
and empyema formation which give rise to foul-smelling sputum.
Treatment of choice is intravenous flucloxacillin.

Q5 a.
Chlamydia pneumonia is commonly seen in individuals in close contact
with infected birds, in particular parrots. Neck stiffness in addition to
photophobia are common occurrences. The treatment of choice includes
tetracycline or erythromycin antibiotics.

Question 3

Q1 f.
This is a classical presentation of tuberculosis. Investigations of choice
include sputum samples for acid-fast bacilli as well as early morning urine
samples. Treatment of choice relies on a quadruple therapy regimen of
rifampicin, isoniazid, pyrazinamide and ethambutol.

Q2 b.
Cystic fibrosis presents with shortness of breath and a dry cough.
Additional features include steatorrhoea due to fat malabsorption, and
infertility. It is an autosomal recessive condition associated with mutation
of the cystic fibrosis transmembrane regulator gene. Diagnosis is made via
the sweat test which demonstrates a sodium and chloride concentration
> 60 mmol/L.

Q3 c.
Chronic obstructive pulmonary disease is commonly seen in long-term
smokers. It is associated with shortness of breath and individuals are at
risk of frequent chest infections. A chest X-ray will often demonstrate
hyperexpanded lung fields. Treatment in an acute setting involves
nebulised bronchodilators and steroids.

Q4 e.
Pulmonary embolism presents with shortness of breath and pleuritic chest
pain. Risk factors include immobility, malignancy, a history of venous
thromboembolism and drugs such as the oral contraceptive pill. The gold
standard investigation of choice is a CTPA. Treatment comprises
enoxaparin 1.5 mg/kg followed by warfarin for 6 months with an
international normalised ratio (INR) of between 2 and 3.

Q5 h.

Pleural effusions present with reduced breath sounds, dullness to percussion and, in some cases, a pleural friction rub. A pleural effusion may be classified as a transudate or exudate. Causes of a transudate include heart failure, cirrhosis and nephrotic syndrome. Examples of an exudate include malignancy, infection and a pulmonary embolus. A pleural effusion is classified as an exudate if it meets any of the following criteria, known as Light's criteria:

Pleural fluid protein/serum protein ratio > 0.5;

Pleural fluid LDH/serum LDH ratio > 0.6;

Pleural fluid LDH more than 2/3 the upper limit of normal for serum LDH.

18 Urology

For each question below, what is the most likely answer?
Select ONE option only from the answers supplied.

1. A 67-year-old man attends his GP for a routine check-up. He comments
   that he has been getting up in the night to pass urine more frequently.
   He also states that he experiences episodes where he feels a sense of
   incomplete emptying. What is the most likely diagnosis?
   a) Ureteric calculi
   b) Urinary tract infection
   c) Benign prostatic hypertrophy
   d) Prostate cancer
   e) Prostatitis

2. A 78-year-old nursing home resident is admitted to hospital. He has a
   background history of mixed vascular and Lewy body dementia.
   He appears confused, stating that one of the nurses hit him and so he
   retaliated by biting her arm. Routine examination proves unremarkable.
   He smells strongly of urine and you note that he has wet the bed.
   A urine dipstick reveals 1+ leucocytes and 1+ nitrites. What is the most
   likely diagnosis?
   a) Benign prostatic hypertrophy
   b) Worsening dementia
   c) Ureteric calculi
   d) Prostate cancer
   e) Urinary tract infection

3. A 34-year-old woman attends her GP. She comments that she has been
   accidentally passing urine when laughing. A routine urine dipstick is
   normal. What is the most likely diagnosis?
   a) Urge incontinence
   b) Stress incontinence

The Complete GPVTS Stage 2 Preparation Guide: Questions and Professional Dilemmas,
First Edition. Edited by Saba Khan with Neel Sharma.
© 2012 John Wiley & Sons, Ltd. Published 2012 by John Wiley & Sons, Ltd.

c) Overflow incontinence

d) Functional incontinence

e) Mixed incontinence

4. A 67-year-old woman presents to her GP. She comments that she has been experiencing the strong need to pass urine and finds it difficult to prevent herself from doing so. What is the most likely diagnosis?
a) Overflow incontinence
b) Mixed incontinence
c) Functional incontinence
d) Urge incontinence
e) Stress incontinence

5. A 69-year-old man presents to his GP for a routine check-up. He comments that he has been accidentally passing urine over the past few weeks. He states that he passes small amounts and has noticed a poor stream during voiding. Past medical history includes type 2 diabetes for which he takes metformin. What is the most likely diagnosis?
a) Stress incontinence
b) Overflow incontinence
c) Functional incontinence
d) Mixed incontinence
e) Urge incontinence

6. A 79-year-old man with severe osteoarthritis of his knees presents to the GP with incontinence. He states that when he needs to pass urine he is unable to make it to the toilet in time and as a result accidentally wets himself. What is the most likely diagnosis?
a) Functional incontinence
b) Urge incontinence
c) Overflow incontinence
d) Mixed incontinence
e) Stress incontinence

7. A 21-year-old man presents to the Emergency Department. He is noted to have a firm scrotal mass which is non-tender on palpation. He states that it does not cause him any pain or discomfort but is worried that it may be something sinister. On further examination you note that the mass does not transilluminate. Routine blood investigations demonstrate an elevated alpha-fetoprotein. What is the most likely diagnosis?
a) Seminoma
b) Epididymal cyst
c) Inguinal hernia
d) Teratoma
e) Testicular torsion

8. A 55-year-old man presents to the GP with a testicular lump. On examination you note a painless firm mass within his right testicle.

Routine blood investigations demonstrate an elevated serum lactate dehydrogenase. What is the most likely diagnosis?
a) Epididymal cyst
b) Testicular torsion
c) Seminoma
d) Inguinal hernia
e) Teratoma

9. A 22-year-old university student presents to the Emergency Department. He complains of pain on passing urine following intercourse. On examination you note he is febrile and has evidence of a yellow-coloured urethral discharge. What is the most likely diagnosis?
a) Urinary tract infection
b) Urethritis
c) Prostatitis
d) Benign prostatic hypertrophy
e) Prostate cancer

10. A 67-year-old man is admitted to hospital following worsening of his chronic obstructive pulmonary disease. He has remained bed-bound since admission and on day 3 he comments that he has not opened his bowels. The nurses inform you that he has been wetting the bed accidentally and prior to admission was continent of urine. Abdominal examination reveals a distended abdomen with scanty bowel sounds. Rectal examination reveals impacted stool. What is the most likely diagnosis?
a) Stress incontinence
b) Transient incontinence
c) Functional incontinence
d) Overflow incontinence
e) Urge incontinence

11. A 35-year-old man presents to the Emergency Department complaining of being unable to pass urine. Abdominal examination reveals lower abdominal tenderness with a palpable bladder. Past medical history includes recurrent urinary tract infections and asthma. A urine dipstick proves normal. What is the most likely diagnosis?
a) Seminoma
b) Urethral stricture
c) Teratoma
d) Prostatitis
e) Urinary tract infection

12. A 62-year-old man attends the Emergency Department with his wife. He complains of increased urinary frequency and urgency. Abdominal examination proves unremarkable. Digital rectal examination reveals a boggy feeling prostate. A urine dipstick is negative. What is the most likely diagnosis?

a) Benign prostatic hypertrophy
b) Urethritis
c) Prostatitis
d Pyelonephritis
e) Urinary tract infection

13. A 14-year-old girl presents to the Emergency Department with sudden-onset left-sided loin pain. On examination you note left flank tenderness. Routine observations demonstrate a temperature of 39.2°C. During the end of your consultation you note she begins to experience rigors. A urine dipstick demonstrates 2+ protein and 2+ leucocytes. What is the most likely diagnosis?
a) Urinary tract infection
b) Pyelonephritis
c) Renal stones
d) Urethral stricture
e) Ectopic pregnancy

14. A 19-year-old male presents with a lump in his scrotum. On examination you note a small swelling which is fluctuant and transilluminates which is separate from the body of the testis. What is the most likely diagnosis?
a) Hydrocele
b) Epididymal cyst
c) Varicocele
d) Teratoma
e) Seminoma

15. A 26-year-old man presents to his GP. He complains of pain in both testicles with urinary dysuria. On examination you note a temperature of 39°C. No masses are palpable in his scrotum. He is in a long-term relationship but recently admitted to being unfaithful during a friend's stag party. What is the most likely diagnosis?
a) Varicocele
b) Teratoma
c) Epididymo-orchitis
d) Inguinal hernia
e) Hydrocele

Extended matching questions

Question 1
a) Benign prostatic hypertrophy
b) Bladder calculi
c) Ureteric calculi
d) Cystitis
e) Bladder cancer
f) Prostate cancer
g) Pyelonephritis
h) Iatrogenic
i) Prostatitis

For each patient below, what is the most likely diagnosis?
Select ONE option only from the list above.
Each option may be selected once, more than once or not at all.

1. An 89-year-old man attends his GP for a routine appointment. He comments that he has noticed blood in his urine over the past 1 week. During voiding he comments that he experiences pain and that he is now passing urine more frequently than normal. He continues to say that he feels generally weak and has lost 2 kg in weight over the past month. Routine blood investigations reveal a urea of 20 mmol/L and a creatinine of 246 μmol/L.
2. A 72-year-old man presents with a 2-day history of painless haematuria. Past medical history includes chronic obstructive pulmonary disease. He continues to smoke and has done so heavily since his early teens. Routine observations reveal a pulse rate of 73 beats per minute, blood pressure of 110/70 mmHg and temperature of 36.5°C. Abdominal, cardiovascular and respiratory examinations prove unremarkable.
3. A 32-year-old man is taken to the Emergency Department by his wife. He complains of severe pain in his right flank which comes in waves. During his assessment he begins to vomit excessive amounts. Past medical history includes ulcerative colitis which is managed with sulphasalazine.
4. A 19-year-old sexually active university student presents with left-sided loin pain radiating to her back. On examination you note evidence of tenderness on palpation on her left side. Routine observations reveal a temperature of 38.5°C.
5. A 60-year-old man presents to his GP with a 1-week history of malaise and lower abdominal discomfort. On further questioning he comments that he has been passing urine more frequently than normal and particularly at night. On examination his abdomen is soft and non-tender. PR examination reveals a tender, boggy prostate. Urine dipstick reveals 1+ protein and 1+ leucocytes.

Question 2
a) Epididymitis
b) Teratoma

c) Hydrocele
d) Inguinal hernia
e) Seminoma
f) Varicocele
g) Haematocele
h) Testicular torsion
i) Bladder cancer

For each patient below, what is the most likely diagnosis?
Select ONE option only from the list above.
Each option may be selected once, more than once or not at all.

1. A 49-year-old male attends his GP with left-sided scrotal swelling. On examination you note enlargement of his left testicle, which feels like a bag of worms and is non-tender on palpation.
2. A 58-year-old man attends his GP clinic with new-onset right-sided scrotal swelling. On examination you note evidence of a soft mass within his scrotum which transilluminates and is fluctuant but non-tender.
3. A 23-year-old gym instructor attends the Emergency Department. He complains of sudden-onset right-sided scrotal pain. During the consultation he begins to vomit profusely. On examination you note the right testicle is extremely tender on palpation and is elevated compared to the left.
4. A 19-year-old boy presents to the Emergency Department with pain in his left testicle after being struck by a football during a local university match. On examination you note evidence of a non-tender lump which is non-translucent and confined to the scrotum. You are unable to identify the testes and epididymis.
5. A 26-year-old man presents to his GP complaining of a four-day history of right-sided scrotal pain and swelling. He comments that it has been difficult to pass urine recently and that he has the desire to pass urine more frequently. On examination you note that elevation of the right scrotum helps to relieve the pain. Routine observations reveal a temperature of 39.2°C.

Question 3
a) Benign prostatic hypertrophy
b) Normal pressure hydrocephalus
c) Urinary tract infection
d) Neurogenic bladder
e) Ureteric stricture
f) Bladder cancer
g) Detrusor instability
h) Prostate cancer
i) Seminoma

For each patient below, what is the most likely diagnosis?
Select ONE option only from the list above.
Each option may be selected once, more than once or not at all.

1. A 72-year-old woman is seen in the urology outpatient clinic. She complains of a two-week history of urinary frequency, nocturia and lower abdominal pain. A routine urine dipstick proves unremarkable. She is referred for urodynamic studies which demonstrate involuntary contraction of her bladder during filling.

2. A 76-year-old woman with a background history of Parkinson's disease presents to the Emergency Department. She complains of difficulty in passing urine and episodes of post-void dribbling. On examination you note evidence of lower abdominal tenderness and a palpable bladder. A urine dipstick proves unremarkable. Routine blood investigations demonstrate normal urea and electrolytes.

3. A 68-year-old man presents with urinary symptoms to his GP. He comments that he has been going to the toilet more frequently at night and that he experiences a sense of incomplete emptying. His wife mentions that he has lost approximately 2 kg in weight over the past 1 week. Abdominal examination proves unremarkable.

4. A 72-year-old man presents to the local urology outpatient clinic following referral by his GP. He comments that he has been finding it difficult to pass urine over the past few days and that his stream is not as strong as compared to a few months back. Blood investigations demonstrate a normal urea and electrolytes. In addition, serum prostate-specific antigen is normal.

5. A 78-year-old woman is admitted to the medical team following being seen in the Emergency Department. The senior house officer who saw her referred the patient on the basis of an abnormal gait and urinary incontinence. A routine urine dipstick demonstrates the presence of 1+ protein, 2+ leucocytes and no nitrites. Her carer who is accompanying her informs you that she has a background history of Alzheimer's dementia.

Answers

Single best answer questions

Q1 c.

Benign prostatic hypertrophy typically presents with increased urinary frequency, nocturia, urgency and a sense of incomplete emptying. Digital rectal examination is essential to rule out possible malignancy. Investigations of importance include urinalysis as well as serum prostate-specific antigen, which is elevated typically in prostate cancer. Treatment of choice includes the use of alpha-1-blockers or 5-alpha reductase inhibitors such as finasteride. Ureteric calculi presents with severe colicky flank pain as well as lower abdominal discomfort. A urinary tract infection is often associated with burning on passing urine as well as haematuria and even a temperature. Prostate cancer, in addition to the urinary symptoms of benign prostatic hypertrophy, also presents with anaemia, weight loss and possibly bone pain secondary to metastases. Prostatitis presents with urinary frequency, dysuria, fever, abdominal pain and general malaise.

Q2 e.

In view of the positive urine dipstick and strong urine odour, the most likely diagnosis is a urinary tract infection. The hallucinations are most likely to be related to his Lewy body dementia which is a hallmark sign of the condition.

Q3 b.

Stress incontinence commonly occurs as a result of increased abdominal pressure secondary to laughing, sneezing and coughing. Pelvic floor muscle weakness is the most common cause of such an occurrence. The treatment of choice includes pelvic floor exercises as well as alpha agonists such as pseudoephedrine.

Q4 d.

This is a typical presentation of urge incontinence. It arises as a result of uninhibited bladder contraction from overactivity of the detrusor muscle. Anticholinergic agents such as oxybutynin and tricyclic antidepressants such as imipramine may prove useful.

Q5 b.

Overflow incontinence typically presents with the accidental passage of small volumes of urine in association with dribbling and a poor stream. It is evident in those with neuropathy, as is the case with diabetes, as well as obstruction such as an enlarged prostate. Alpha-blockers are the mainstay form of treatment.

Q6 a.

Functional incontinence is seen in individuals with normal urinary systems but with physical or psychological factors that often impair them from reaching the toilet in sufficient time. Treatment of the underlying cause is beneficial.

Q7 d.

A teratoma presents as a painless firm mass in the scrotum. They are often seen in children and young adults. It is important to test the levels of serum alpha-fetoprotein and beta-hCG, which are often elevated. The treatment of choice involves orchidectomy. A seminoma is also painless but associated with an elevated lactate dehydrogenase. An epididymal cyst will present as a fluctuant mass which transilluminates. An inguinal hernia is associated with a swelling above and medial to the pubic tubercle. Testicular torsion results in sudden-onset severe unilateral scrotal pain.

Q8 c.

This is a typical presentation of a seminoma, which is often associated with an elevated serum lactate dehydrogenase. Treatment involves the use of external beam radiotherapy, chemotherapy or surgery.

Q9 b.

This is a classic presentation of urethritis secondary to sexual intercourse. Antibiotics are the mainstay form of management.

Q10 b.

Transient incontinence is often seen in hospitalised patients and can occur secondary to confusion, infection, stool impaction and reduced mobility. Treatment of the underlying cause helps to resolve the incontinence.

Q11 b.

Urethral strictures are usually caused by trauma or secondary to recurrent urinary tract infections or renal calculi. The treatment of choice is typically surgical.

Q12 c.

Prostatitis presents with fever and urinary symptoms including urgency, frequency and dysuria. Treatment of choice includes antibiotics, typically doxycycline or ciprofloxacin.

Q13 b.

Pyelonephritis typically presents with fever, lower abdominal pain and flank discomfort. Management involves the use of intravenous fluids, analgesia and antibiotics such as ceftriaxone or gentamicin.

Q14 b.

This is a typical presentation of an epididymal cyst. A hydrocele is a soft, non-tender swelling which also transilluminates. It is differentiated from an epididymal cyst in that the testes and epididymis are not able to be identified. A varicocele is often palpable and described as feeling like a bag of worms.

Q15 c.
Symptoms include testicular pain and fevers seen commonly after unprotected sexual intercourse. Analgesia and antibiotics are the treatment of choice. In case of abscess formation, surgical drainage may be indicated.

Extended matching questions
Question 1
Q1 f.
Prostate cancer presents with haematuria and weight loss as well as urinary urgency and frequency. Rectal examination may demonstrate a hard palpable prostate. Blood investigations of importance include serum urea and creatinine as well as prostate-specific antigen which is often elevated. Treatment of choice includes surgery or radiotherapy. For metastatic disease, LHRH analogues and anti-androgens are useful.

Q2 e.
Bladder cancer presents with painless haematuria. Smoking and other carcinogenic agents such as nitrosamine are common aetiological agents. For non-invasive disease, intravesical chemotherapy or surgery are the main forms of treatment. For invasive disease, chemotherapy alone is useful.

Q3 c.
Ureteric calculi present with nausea, vomiting and flank pain. Causes include hyperparathyroidism, hyperuricaemia, bacterial infection, diets high in purine-containing foods such as fish and legumes, as well as certain drugs such as sulphasalazine and magnesium-based antacids. Fluid resuscitation, analgesia, antibiotics and alpha-blockers are proven to be effective.

Q4 g.
This is a classic presentation of pyelonephritis. Treatment of choice includes antibiotics, analgesia and fluids.

Q5 i.
Typical symptoms include fever, malaise, abdominal pain as well as urinary frequency and urgency. Treatment of choice involves the use of antibiotics and fluids.

Question 2
Q1 f.
A varicocele arises as a result of dilatation of the pampiniform venous plexus and internal spermatic vein. Treatment of choice is surgical intervention.

Q2 c.
A hydrocele arises as a result of fluid collection within the tunica vaginalis of the scrotum. Management is surgical.

Q3 h.
Testicular torsion arises as a result of a congenital anomaly, trauma or excessive exercise. It is typically observed in those below the age of 30 and results in impaired blood flow to the testicle. Treatment is based on the use of analgesia and surgical intervention.

Q4 g.
A haematocele is a collection of blood in the tunica vaginalis and occurs typically after a traumatic injury. It is distinguished from a hydrocele as it does not transilluminate.

Q5 a.
Acute epididymitis presents following bacterial or viral infection and is commonly seen after sexual intercourse. Treatment of choice involves the use of analgesia and antibiotics.

Question 3
Q1 g.
Detrusor instability is diagnosed following urodynamic studies which demonstrate involuntary bladder contraction. Treatment of choice involves the use of anticholinergic agents such as oxybutynin and tolterodine.

Q2 d.
Neurogenic bladder presents with symptoms of overflow incontinence. It can arise as a result of a stroke, spinal injury, Parkinson's disease, multiple sclerosis or vitamin B12 deficiency. Research suggests the use of catheterisation and increased fluid intake as a form of management.

Q3 h.
Prostate cancer presents with urinary frequency, nocturia and a sense of incomplete emptying post-voiding as well as weight loss and haematuria. Serum prostate-specific antigen is typically elevated. The treatment of choice involves the use of radiotherapy and surgery. Hormonal-based agents such as LHRH analogues are useful for metastatic disease.

Q4 a.
This is a classic presentation of benign prostatic hypertrophy. Treatment of choice involves the use of alpha-blockers. An elevated serum prostate-specific antigen in addition to weight loss should raise alarm bells to the possibility of malignant transformation.

Q5 b.
Normal pressure hydrocephalus is associated with urinary incontinence, an ataxic gait and dementia. It arises as a result of distortion of the corona radiata by the distended ventricles. Management involves the use of surgical intervention in the form of cerebrospinal fluid shunting.

Part 2
Professional Dilemmas

19 Ranking Questions

The following questions have been written in the format of the first type of question that you may encounter in the exam. The candidate must read the scenario and then rank the options A to E in order of most appropriate (A) to least appropriate (E). It is best to attempt all questions as there are no negative marks awarded for these questions.

1. You are at the GP surgery and are coming toward the end of your attachment. One of your patients has been seeing you regularly for a skin problem that you helped to resolve. They leave you a gift of one hundred pounds as a gesture of thanks.
   What action do you take?
   A Donate it into the practice fund to be shared equally.
   B Keep it and don't declare it.
   C Feel offended and ask the secretary to return it.
   D Contact the patient to say thank you and to make sure there has been no misunderstanding before deciding what to do with the gift.
   E Give it to your educational supervisor as he is the patient's named doctor.

2. You are completing a rotation in Obstetrics and Gynaecology. You are asked to obtain consent from a female patient for sterilisation. You are happy to do this in theory as you have read all about the procedure but you have not seen it done.
   What is the best course of action?
   A You ask a senior colleague for more information on the procedure prior to seeing the patient.
   B You discuss the procedure with your registrar and ask them if they will go with you to carry out the consent procedure to make sure that all the patient's concerns are addressed.
   C Go to the patient and complete the consent paperwork while trying to guess the answers to most of their questions.
   D Leave it for someone else to do as you do not feel qualified for the task.

The Complete GPVTS Stage 2 Preparation Guide: Questions and Professional Dilemmas, First Edition. Edited by Saba Khan with Neel Sharma.
© 2012 John Wiley & Sons, Ltd. Published 2012 by John Wiley & Sons, Ltd.

    E Ask your colleague who is also a foundation trainee to go with you as you do not want to look incompetent to the patient or your team.

3. A 23-year-old patient who has previously enjoyed private healthcare comes into hospital overnight because of back pain. On history and examination there are no red flag signs and no features suggestive of serious underlying causes. A diagnosis of mechanical back pain is made and the patient is advised that she can go home. The patient refuses and insists that she should be kept in a room overnight and reviewed by the consultant in the morning.

   Rank the following responses in order.

   A Tell her to go home and stop wasting valuable hospital resources.

   B Advise her that there is no way she can be seen by the consultant as she does not have any serious health issues, but that she can go home and see her GP the following day.

   C Advise her that you can call a more senior member of your team to give her a second opinion and allay her concerns about her condition. Document all discussion and examination findings in the notes.

   D Admit her to stop her causing a fuss and carry on with your busy workload, and let your senior deal with her when they have time.

   E Advise her that you will call and discuss her case with the most senior member of your team available to ensure that you have not missed anything.

4. A 46-year-old patient with depression presents to you, a trainee while on a GP attachment. The patient has decided that they don't want to take their antidepressants any more as they feel aromatherapy is a better option. They have a history of deliberate self-harm during previous bouts of severe depression.

   Please order these responses from A to E, with A being the most suitable and E being the least suitable.

   A Ask your trainer to see him as you cannot deal with the confrontation.

   B Advise the patient of the risks and benefits of his previous drug treatment, and discuss his reasons for wanting to change. Advise him that best practice for his condition is to use regular medication as there is insufficient evidence to support the use of aromatherapy.

   C Agree with the patient and when they have left arrange a mental health assessment.

   D Discuss the treatment options and then agree that if aromatherapy is the option he wishes to try then it is his choice.

   E Tell the patient that aromatherapy is nonsense and that he must listen to your advice on treatment of his condition.

5. You are working at a practice and one of the trainers comes into your room to help you with some paperwork. You find that he smells strongly of alcohol, but is due to start a surgery shortly. He has had

several complaints recently, one of which you are aware of as it was discussed as a 'significant event'.

Order the following responses in order of most appropriate to least appropriate.

A You are worried about telling anyone as it is only a suspicion and you have no evidence to support your claim, so you say nothing.

B You go and speak to the reception staff as they are easy to talk to and have been very friendly since you started your rotation. They also seem to know how to deal with most things.

C You ring the GMC and report the doctor.

D You ring the GMC and discuss the case for advice without giving his details, and then also speak to your defence union as another source of information.

E You discuss your concerns with your own trainer and ask them to deal with it.

6. A 15-year-old girl presents to you at the GP surgery while you are there on rotation. She has asked to see you alone as she urgently needs to see someone. She requests the pill, and tells you she is sexually active with her 15-year-old boyfriend. Her parents are unaware of the relationship and she has not told them of her visit to the doctor.

Order your responses in the most appropriate order.

A Advise the patient that she should abstain as she is under age and that you refuse to give her the pill.

B Ask her to come back with her mother as you refuse to prescribe her the pill without her mother present.

C Assess her understanding of contraceptive options, the side effects and outcome of treatment. Ensure that she is aware that barrier methods are still required to prevent STIs and then prescribe.

D Call social services as this is a child protection issue as she is underage.

E Discuss her case with the receptionist whose daughter is at the same school and might know more about the patient.

7. You are a new doctor on the ward, and have recently started to take more responsibility within the team. On one particular morning you are asked to discharge whichever patients you feel are able to go home as the registrar is off sick and the consultant is busy in clinic.

Order the following responses as appropriate.

A You work your way through to the best of your ability and discharge those patients that you feel are probably ok to go home.

B You see all the patients but discharge none of them as you are too worried about making a mistake.

C You see the patients but ask the on-call registrar to review your discharges whenever they have time.

D You go and see medical staffing and ask them to arrange senior cover as you do not feel comfortable with the responsibility and do not wish to compromise patient safety.

E Discharge as many patients as possible to impress the team when they return.

8. A patient presents to you while you are completing a GP rotation. She is 49 years old and speaks very little English. From what you can understand she is having difficulty in her marriage and is feeling low. You arrange for her to return with an interpreter. On arrival one of the reception staff recognises the interpreter as a relative of the patient. Arrange the responses appropriately.

A Carry on with the consultation and ignore the fact that confidentiality is an issue, as it has taken so much work to organise the consultation and you want to address the problem as soon as possible.

B Ask the interpreter to wait outside and just try and muddle through with the patient.

C Take the patient aside and ask her if she is happy with the interpreter, and only proceed if she is happy and you are satisfied she has made an informed decision.

D See the patient but skirt over any uncomfortable questions to avoid embarrassment.

E Rearrange the appointment after explaining confidentiality issues with the interpreter.

9. You are nearing the end of your rotation at the hospital and you are approached by a patient. They tell you how much they appreciate your support and treatment, and ask you if you would join them for dinner after work one evening.
Order the following responses in the most appropriate way.

A You consider what to do and feel it would be rude to refuse, so you agree to go but with another colleague.

B You don't feel it is appropriate as the patient has only just been discharged; you agree to meet in a few weeks.

C You do not feel it is appropriate as a professional relationship should be maintained even if the patient is discharged.

D You consult your senior as you are unsure of what is best practice as you do not want to upset the patient.

E You agree as you see nothing wrong with going as the patient has been discharged.

10. You see an 18-year-old girl while on attachment at the surgery. She advises you that her partner is abusive and has been hitting her over the last few months. She has an 11-month-old baby living with her. She reassures you that her partner has never hit the child. She does not want to leave him.
Order the following responses appropriately.

A Explain to the patient that you are duty bound to report the case to child protection services as her child could be at risk of abuse.

B Tell the patient to leave her partner and seek help or you will report the case.

C Do nothing as she has said that she does not wish to leave, and has reassured you that the child is unharmed.

D Give her written information and explain avenues for help. Ask her to return to discuss things further.

E Call the police as a crime has been committed and you are duty bound to report abuse to the appropriate authorities.

11. You are an F2 doctor and are 2 weeks into your new job. You are aware that oral morphine went missing from your ward a few months ago, and apparently this was not the first time. Rumours have been circulating that one of the nurses is responsible, and that she may be self-medicating. On starting your shift you notice the nurse in question removing two morphine vials from the controlled drug cupboard without signing for them. This is not witnessed by anyone else.
Rank in order from A to E the following actions in response to this situation.

A Fill out an IR1 (Incident Record) form as per hospital protocol.

B Do nothing as you have only been at the hospital for a few weeks and you do not want to create undue tension with colleagues.

C Try to speak to your registrar, who is currently stuck in theatre with a difficult case and won't be available for several hours.

D Wait and discuss the situation at your next appraisal meeting.

E Immediately ask to speak to the nurse in question privately to discuss your concerns, away from the ward and other staff members.

12. You are in the middle of a ward round when one of the patients asks if they can speak to you in private. You agree to do so and they inform you that their mobile phone is missing.
Rank in order the following actions in response to this situation.

A Tell the patient he must have misplaced his phone and that it will turn up.

B Comfort the patient regarding the theft. Get a detailed description of the item, and a detailed account of when he saw it last.

C Ascertain the details of the alleged theft, and then inform the nurse in charge to call the police.

D Ask other patients on the ward if they have seen the phone and then start a search of patients' bedside lockers.

E Fill out a critical incident form.

13. One of your colleagues has been consistently calling in sick, especially during on-call commitments at weekends. Last weekend when you were on call, he called in sick and they were unable to find a locum at such short notice. You find out, however, that during these absences

from work he is actually working as a locum at another hospital. What do you do?

Rank in order the following actions in response to this situation.

A Inform the GMC.

B Speak to your colleague directly and inform him that what he is doing is wrong and that if he continues in this way you will need to inform your seniors.

C Do nothing; you do not want to be the bearer of bad news.

D Tell your consultant immediately.

E Go and speak to medical staffing and let them know what has been going on.

14. You are a senior house officer and are on call for general medicine. The other senior house officer on call with you seems to be making inappropriate decisions, as you have been bleeped all night to come and correct his prescriptions or re-review patients that he has already seen.

Rank in order the following actions in response to this situation.

A Contact your registrar immediately and inform him of your concerns.

B Find the other senior house officer and challenge his decisions in front of other members of staff. Ask him to explain himself and tell him why he is wrong.

C Inform your registrar that you are going home. You are not going to do the jobs of two doctors as he is clearly incompetent.

D Contact medical staffing and ask them to find a replacement.

E Say nothing. It is not up to you to decide that he is not doing his job properly.

15. You are on call at night and are bleeped to the ward to review an elderly patient with known Alzheimer's dementia. When you arrive the patient in question is walking around the ward quietly, not causing any harm to himself or other patients. The nurse in charge demands that you sedate him, as she insists the patient is being both physically and verbally aggressive.

Rank in order the following actions in response to this situation.

A Explain to the nursing staff that you do not feel it appropriate to sedate this gentleman when he is fully mobile and not, from your assessment, causing harm to anyone. Explain that you appreciate how it may be difficult for the night staff to manage but that you will ensure that the patient's behaviour as reported by the nurse during the night is duly documented and discussed with his team in the morning.

B Discuss the patient with the registrar to see what he feels is appropriate.

C Refuse to sedate the patient, based on the grounds that it is unnecessary. Remind the nursing staff that they are there to nurse the patients, and as long as he is not a danger to himself it is their job to simply keep an eye on him.

D Sedate the patient as you do not want to get on the nurse's bad side.

E Try to encourage the patient to go back to bed and sit with him until he settles.

16. You have just finished having dinner and decide to take a taxi home. You note that the taxi driver is in fact a patient of yours. He had recently been diagnosed with epilepsy over a week ago and had been informed he should no longer drive as a result. He has an appointment to see you in clinic next week.

Rank in order the following actions in response to this situation.

A Say nothing whatsoever as you tend to not get taxis often anyway.

B Inform him again that he should not be driving and that he should contact the DVLA. Try to find out why he is still driving and make him understand the gravity of the issue.

C Explain to him that, as you know he is still driving and has ignored all medical advice, you have no choice but to inform the DVLA.

D Berate him in a bid to stop him driving.

E Phone his wife and tell her that her husband is still driving and see if she can stop him.

17. You are on call over the weekend. You meet the night senior house officer for handover and notice he looks rather unkempt. You are certain you can smell alcohol on his breath and notice an empty half-bottle of vodka in the bin. What do you do?

Rank in order the following actions in response to this situation.

A Say nothing as it is of no concern to yourself.

B Speak to your colleague immediately and in private. Ask him if he has been drinking at work and if so ask what you can do to help him.

C Speak to the nursing staff to see if they have noticed that he appeared drunk overnight.

D Report him to the GMC as a matter of urgency.

E Discuss the matter with your registrar.

18. A 19-year-old girl attends her GP for a repeat contraceptive pill prescription. During the consultation you note some unusual bruising to her arms. On further questioning she breaks down in tears and informs you that she has had a recent argument with her boyfriend, who assaulted her. She tells you that she does not want to take the matter forward and is just grateful that she has been able to talk to someone about the situation. What would you do?

Rank in order the following actions in response to this situation.

A Phone the police as she has been assaulted and her boyfriend should be arrested.

B Document everything very clearly including her injuries and her account of what happened with her boyfriend.

C Do nothing as she has stated that she does not want to take the matter further.

D Advise her that it is really up to her if she wants to take this matter further. Inform her that support groups are available and the procedures that are in place if she chooses to report the assault at a later date.

E Contact her boyfriend, who is also your patient, and tell him that his behaviour is unacceptable and that if it happens again you will report him to the police.

19. You have left work over an hour ago and are on the way to a wedding reception when you realise that you did not write up warfarin for a patient. You try to phone the F2 doctor on call but are unable to get through. What do you do?

Rank in order the following actions in response to this situation.

A Do nothing as you suspect the nurses will realise that you have not written up the drug and will get someone else to do it.

B Go to the wedding reception and call again later.

C Call the ward and inform the nurse in charge that the patient does not have warfarin written up and can the on-call doctor be bleeped to prescribe it.

D Call the specialist registrar to write up the warfarin and explain that you have been unable to contact the F2 doctor on call.

E Go back to the hospital, write up the warfarin yourself and be late for the wedding reception.

20. You are called to review a patient who has spiked a temperature. When you review the patient you note that they are halfway through a course of intravenous amoxicillin. As you document your assessment in the notes you realise that the patient is in fact allergic to penicillin. What do you do?

Rank in order the following actions in response to this situation.

A Say nothing, they have already had a few days of amoxicillin with no harm caused.

B Tell the sister in charge and ask her to stop the infusion immediately.

C Explain to the patient what has happened. Be honest and open. Apologise and be empathetic.

D Do nothing but fill out an IR1 form as per hospital protocol.

E Tell the patient that you feel they are not responding as well as you would expect them to with the antibiotic prescribed; as such you will change them to another one which is non-penicillin-based.

Answers

Q1 D, A, E, B, C.

Option D is the best option as it will clear up any possible misunderstandings, and can then also be logged in the notes as patient contact.

Option A would allow everyone to benefit and show that you appreciate the teamworking aspect that is so important to both training and practising as a qualified practitioner.

In option E, your supervisor is a good person to turn to and if you felt that he was more deserving of the gift then you could give it to him, though the gift was given to you by the patient and was therefore meant for your benefit.

In option B, keeping the gift and not telling anyone would open up issues around probity within your own practice and ethics as a doctor. Financial gifts should be declared and recorded to avoid later confusion.

Option C is the least desirable option as it would probably offend the patient and cause longer-term problems for the practice. Also asking the secretary to return it is unfair, as it would put them in a difficult position.

Q2 B, A, E, C, D.

Option B is the best response, as the patient may have questions that you cannot address. The registrar will have completed the procedure or assisted in one and therefore is better placed to describe how the procedure is carried out.

Option A allows you to find out more about the specific procedure in question and therefore to have more information to give the patient. However you still may have knowledge gaps, given that you have never seen the procedure.

Option E shows that you have asked for help but from the least experienced member of the team, which is not in the best interest of the patient.

In option C you are completing the task but not offering the patient the choice of seeing someone who could address their concerns better.

Option D is the least desirable option as it is not dealing with the issue and could cause the patient to have a delay in their procedure if the necessary paperwork is not completed.

Q3 C, E, B, D, A.

Option C is the best of these options as it addresses the patient's concerns and also ensures that nothing has been missed. Careful documentation is important in the event that something has been missed and also if a complaint is made.

Option E is also involving a more senior member of the team, and also ensures that the patient's interest is put first regardless of the clinician's opinion.

Option B is not a very professional way to deal with the patient as it does not address patient choice and is ignoring the patient's wishes. It does, however, offer a safety net by advising her to seek a second opinion the following day.

Option D is a less suitable option, as it is a misuse of hospital resources and is also shifting the responsibility to another clinician without discussion.

Option A is rude and unprofessional and would not be in keeping with good medical practice. Patients are entitled to a second opinion within reason and should also have their concerns addressed in the event that something has been missed. As a junior clinician it is not reasonable to take this course of action as it could have more serious repercussions for the responsible team.

Q4 B, D, E, A, C.
Option B is the most suitable option as it addresses the patient's choice but also utilises the advisory role of a clinician.

Option D is a less preferable choice as, although it is presenting treatment options, there is no recommendation for the best option for him, which is less in line with good practice.

Option E is not addressing patient choice at all, and therefore is a less suitable answer. Patient autonomy is an important ethical consideration in any consultation and therefore should always be respected.

Option A takes responsibility away from you as a doctor, and would not allow you to develop your own ability to deal with patients who wish to use different treatment options to those that are considered best practice. As a clinician it is important to be able to deal with patient choice and confrontation in a professional and appropriate way.

For option C, the Mental Health Act can only be applied in cases where the patient is not deemed to be competent. In this case the patient has a different opinion, but is completely aware of his choice and is choosing to not adhere to treatment.

Q5 D, C, E, B, A.
Option D would allow you to gain the most correct advice in the given situation and also would mean that you are directly actioning your concerns. Once you have discussed the case, you may be advised that the case can be dealt with locally, in which event the correct procedure for this will be explained to you.

Option C is harsh but is still making sure that something is done and is protecting patient safety.

In option E, asking your trainer to deal with things is taking responsibility away from you, which is easy but not best practice. However, it is still a positive action as you are asking for help and dealing with the concern.

Option B is is not a good option as your concerns are not proven and the reception staff are not best placed to deal with probity issues. It is also a destructive thing to do in a small working environment.

Option A, doing nothing, is the least desirable option as you have not addressed the issue and patient safety could be an issue.

Q6 C, B, A, D, E.
Option C assesses her competence and hence allows you to make a clinical judgement as to whether or not she understands the treatment and if she is aware of the side effects. If you feel she understands the treatment and can make a reasoned judgement, then prescribing for her will ensure that she is safe and also feels able to access healthcare when needed.

With option B, it is good practice to involve family members in patients that are underage. However, this can only be done with the patient's consent and for their best interest. It is however a less appropriate response as it is not treating her immediate need.

Option A is an unrealistic option and also sends a poor message to the patient, showing healthcare to be inaccessible and is not putting her interests first.

For option D, the patient is underage as is her partner; however, in this situation where the relationship is consensual, social services rarely become involved.

Option E is the worst option as it is breaking confidentiality and also unprofessional.

Q7 D, C, B, A, E.
Option D allows you to find suitable cover for your team and also is putting patient safety first as well as alerting the hospital to existing practice that is perhaps inappropriate.

Option C is also ensuring patient safety, however there is a risk that some patients may be discharged prior to the registrar seeing them.

Option B is not a useful way to work as no decisions will be made; however, patient safety should not be directly compromised.

Option A is not the best option as you may be complying with your team's wishes but there is an issue of patient safety which must be addressed.

Option E is poor practice and would compromise patient care.

Q8 C, E, B, D, A.
Option C is the best solution as it allows you to still see the patient if she is happy but also addresses the issue of confidentiality head on.

Option E also addresses the confidentiality issue but does not give the patient a chance to voice her opinion.

Option B prevents breaking confidentiality but would potentially miss serious issues with the patient, and hence could risk patient safety.

Option D would potentially miss any issues of abuse or mental health problems. Also it would be difficult to assess suicide risk if needed.

Option A is the least desirable option as it may miss serious issues as the patient is afraid to disclose information and is also potentially breaking confidentiality.

Q9 C, D, A, B, E.

Option C is the best answer. GMC guidance states that it would be inappropriate to have any kind of relationship with a patient, even after they have been discharged from your care as this is the best way to maintain professionalism.

Option D is a good option. When in doubt as a junior member of staff, it is always appropriate to ask for help and guidance. In this instance you would be given experienced advice, however if still in doubt, guidance can be sought from the GMC and also from your defence body.

Option A is not best practice as it could still potentially compromise you, however the chaperone would be helpful.

Options B and E are the worst options. Informal contact with patients is considered unprofessional, regardless of the time frame.

Q10 A, D, B, C, E.

Option A is the most appropriate option in this case as the child is in a home where domestic abuse is taking place. In this situation there is a risk of abuse to the child, as abuse is categorised as sexual, physical, mental and neglect. Child protection services would then make their own appropriate investigations to ensure that the child is not at risk. It is good practice when duty bound to break confidentiality to inform the patient in order to maintain the long-term relationship.

Option D also addresses the abuse issue and also opens up the opportunity to revisit the discussion at another time. However, there is no guarantee that she would return and the child could be at risk in the interim period.

Option B is coercive which is unprofessional. The patient's choice to stay with her partner is ultimately her choice and this should have no bearing on your duty of care to her child.

Option C is a weak response and does not address care of the patient or her child.

Option E is the worst choice. The police are not the correct avenue in this case as they are duty bound to only act in cases where there is immediate risk or if there is evidence for previous abuse. The patient would also be needed to explain her case. As a clinician it is our role to highlight suspicion of abuse to child protection services so as to allow them to investigate in an appropriate and sensitive manner.

Q11 E, C, A, D, B.

The nurse is stealing controlled drugs which is highly illegal. She is also a risk to the safety of patients on the ward if she is self-medicating. Your first priority should be to the patient. Option E is the only option that gives you an immediate beneficial action.

Option C, speaking to your registrar, is the next best option.

Option A, filling out an IR1 form, would be the next best option as the matter will be formally reported and acted upon. However, the time frame is not ideal as it can take up to a month for such matters to be investigated.

Option D, namely waiting to your next appraisal, also addresses the issue but at a much later time scale than options E, C and A. Appraisal meetings are usually a few months apart and the nurse in question is likely to continue being a danger to patients on the ward.

Option B, doing nothing, is the least appropriate option as you are turning a blind eye and compromising patient safety significantly.

Q12 B, C, E, D, A.

This question is assessing your empathy and communication skills but also how you solve the problem in the question.

Option A is the least appropriate action as you are ignoring the problem entirely as well as indirectly implying that the patient is not speaking the truth.

Options B and C both involve you getting an account of what happened, allowing you to verify the facts. However, option B is a more appropriate option than C as the former demonstrates strong patient empathy.

Option C is the next most appropriate option as it allows you to get the necessary details regarding the theft so that the police can be notified.

Option E would be the third most appropriate action. Although it does not involve taking immediate action it ensures the theft is highlighted to higher management who will act upon it swiftly and appropriately.

Option D whereby you question the other ward patients and perform a locker search is not the best option. Although it does involve immediate action, you are making the theft public to the entire ward, and by searching all the lockers you are demonstrating a lack of trust in your patients which would have profound effects on the doctor–patient relationship model. In addition, by making the theft known to the ward you may induce considerable distress to the patients. Hence D is the fourth option.

Q13 B, D, E, A, C.

Option C is the least suitable option, as this involves you doing nothing, which does not tackle the problem directly.

Option A is the next least suitable option here. It is not appropriate to inform the GMC. Informing the GMC is the last resort and only if the matter has not been solved locally.

Option B is the most appropriate option as it involves immediately tackling the problem in a professional fashion. It allows you to let your colleague know that you are aware of what he is doing, but also gives him an opportunity to explain himself.

This leaves options D and E. Both of these options involve you speaking to someone more senior. It would be more appropriate to raise your concerns with your consultant rather to approach medical staffing as your consultant is directly responsible for your training and welfare.

Q14 A, D, B, E, C.
Options A and D are the best options as they immediately deal with the issue at hand. Speaking to your registrar is the most suitable option as he is in a position to assess the patients seen and to see if there is indeed a problem with the other senior house officer's management. He is also in a better position to contact medical staffing and send home the other senior house officer if needed in order to ensure patient safety is not compromised.

Option B would be the third best option. It ensures that action is taken but without courtesy or sympathy to the senior house officer involved.

Options E and C involve doing nothing whatsoever. Option E is more appropriate than option C as the latter will result in your registrar being left without a full team, hence impairing the mechanics of the on-call shift and compromising patient safety by leaving a senior house officer in charge who is clearly not safe to continue working.

Q15 E, B, A, C, D.
The patient is wandering happily and is causing no harm to himself or others. As such, sedating him is completely inappropriate and would be unethical. Hence option D is the least appropriate action. The most appropriate option is E, whereby you go to see the patient and try to get him back to bed.

Option B is the second best option as you are recognising that you do not deem the sedation appropriate but recognise that the nursing staff feel the patient is difficult to handle. By asking the registrar for advice you are taking an immediate action of seeking senior support.

Option A is the third best option as you are explaining your reasoning behind not wanting to sedate the patient in a polite and professional manner, while also taking on the concerns of your colleagues.

Option C is the second least favourable option as you are interacting with fellow staff members in a disrespectful fashion. You are demonstrating poor communication skills as well as poor team working skills.

Q16 B, C, E, D, A.

The least suitable option is A as you are ignoring the problem at hand.

Option B is the most suitable option as you are communicating your concern with the patient again and explaining why it has serious implications not only for him but for the general public.

Option C is the next suitable option as you are allowed to break patient confidentiality if it is in the public's best interests. You are also informing the patient that you are going to do this.

Option E is the third best option as, although you are breaking confidentiality, you are ensuring his wife is aware of the situation.

Option D, whereby you berate him for what he is doing, will no doubt hinder the doctor–patient relationship and therefore is less suitable than E.

Q17 B, E, C, D, A.

The best option is to discuss the incident there and then with your colleague hence option B is the most appropriate.

The next most suitable option is E, discussing it with your registrar. It ensures that someone senior is aware of what has happened and they will inform you of the next most appropriate steps to take.

Option C is not a favourable option as it involves discussing the incident with other workers which could cause potential damage to the credibility of the senior house officer concerned.

Option D, reporting the incident direct to the GMC, is the next least suitable option. Despite your suspicions you have no concrete proof that he has been drinking and hence it would be inappropriate to inform the GMC at this stage.

Option A is the least suitable option as it involves ignoring what has happened completely.

Q18 D, B, C, A, E.

Option D is the most appropriate option. She has confided in you as her doctor and hence it is your responsibility to offer her the appropriate support and inform her of the possible options available to her.

Option B is the next best option as she may well change her mind in the future and choose to press charges.

Option E is the least suitable option as you are breaking the patient's confidentiality and may as a result put her at more harm.

This leaves us with options A and C. C is the more suitable option as it does not involve you breaking confidentiality. She has stated that she does not want to take this matter further and hence you have a duty to respect her wishes.

Q19 D, C, B, E, A.

Option A is the least suitable option as it involves ignoring the problem at hand.

Option E is the second least suitable option. At first glance it seems appropriate but the working hours of junior doctors are governed in accordance to the European Working Time Directive whereby handing over to colleagues is essential if not all jobs have been achieved within the hours contracted. Hence to return to the hospital when you have already left some time ago is not a worthwhile option.

With regard to options C and D, D is the most appropriate option as you are handing over the warfarin prescription to your senior who will ensure the job is not forgotten. Option C is the next suitable choice as it ensures that the nurse will bleep the on-call doctor currently on site to prescribe the patient's warfarin. This leaves option B as the third choice.

Q20 B, C, E, D, A.

Options D and A are least suitable as they involve you doing nothing about the current antibiotic that is prescribed and as such the patient's condition is at risk. Of the two options, A involves you doing nothing at all and hence is the least suitable.

Option B involves you stopping the drug immediately and making other staff members aware of the problem, so this is the most suitable option.

Option C involves you talking openly and honestly, accepting responsibility for the mistake and showing empathy to the patient, so this is the next best option.

Option E does involve you stopping the medication, so you are removing any form of potential harm being caused to the patient. However, you are being dishonest to the patient and misleading them with regard to what has happened, which is not in keeping with the duties of a good doctor.

20 Multiple Best Answer Questions

This is the second format of question that you may encounter in the professional dilemma section. The candidate must again read the scenario but then decide from the five or more options given (in this case, options A to E) which three would be most appropriate in response to the dilemma described. There is no ranking of the three options. In these questions there are key answers that are correct; however, if candidates choose another option that is 'less correct', they would still be awarded some marks though not as many as for the key answer. For the purposes of this text the three most appropriate 'key' options are given in the answer section.

1. You are an F2 doctor on your first shift in surgery when you are bleeped at 3 am to attend a patient who has had a laparotomy. The wound has completely dehisced and you note the patient's bowel has protruded outside the abdominal cavity. You have never handled this kind of situation before and you feel it is completely outside your level of competence.
   Which three of the following would you pick as your best course of action?
   A Refuse to go and see the patient.
   B Ask the nurses to contact the patient's family as you are concerned about his current state.
   C Assess the patient as best you can, ensuring they are as stable as possible.
   D Ask the nurses to bleep the registrar to inform him about the unwell patient.
   E Tell the nursing staff that you will be there shortly, but go and do other jobs, hoping they will appreciate how busy you are.

2. Your consultant has recently separated from his wife. Since the separation you have noticed a significant change in his behaviour. He is often upset at work, and easy to anger, and occasionally irrational in clinical judgement. You note that he arrives late to work and leaves early. You have noticed that he is making some obvious errors, in

The Complete GPVTS Stage 2 Preparation Guide: Questions and Professional Dilemmas, First Edition. Edited by Saba Khan with Neel Sharma.
© 2012 John Wiley & Sons, Ltd. Published 2012 by John Wiley & Sons, Ltd.

particular with drug prescriptions, whereby he recently prescribed a patient paracetamol and penicillin for a chest infection despite the patient being allergic to both medications. Which three of the following would you pick as your best course of action?

A Call the General Medical Council (GMC) and discuss with them your concerns.

B Say nothing; he is obviously going through a rough time with the separation. Once he has time to acclimatise he will be back to his usual self.

C Remain vigilant with regards to your consultant's behaviour.

D Speak with a senior colleague who is likely to be impartial about your concerns, and get their advice.

E Fill out an incident form with regard to the prescribing errors that have occurred.

3. You are on call and are covering all the medical wards. You are bleeped by a nurse as two family members of a patient are demanding to speak to a doctor. You do not know the patient and have not been involved in her care. The nurse informs you that the family are very angry about the care their mother is receiving. In addition you overhear one of the relatives shouting in the background as to why her mother has not been moved to the local hospice as previously decided.

Which three of the following would you pick as your best course of action?

A Inform the family that you will do your best to answer their questions using their mother's medical notes.

B Speak to the family and inform them that if they want to make a complaint regarding their mother's care then you can give them a copy of the complaints procedure.

C Speak to the family in person rather than ignoring their presence.

D Continue the conversation with the nurse over the phone as long as possible in the hope that the family will get tired of waiting and will go home.

E Inform the family that you are not familiar with their mother's case directly.

F Ask the family to leave the ward as you are busy.

G Ask the family to read the notes themselves as you do not know the patient at all.

4. You are called in the middle of the night to assess a 90-year-old man who has not passed urine. He has a catheter in situ and has only passed 100 mL in the last 24 hours. On review you see that this man's oral intake has been poor for the last 4–5 days and he has had no intravenous fluids prescribed. You prescribe him intravenous normal saline at a 2-hourly rate after inserting a cannula into his right arm. You return to review him after 90 minutes to find that his fluids are still not running. Which three of the following would you pick as your best course of action?

A Stay on the ward until you are sure that the fluids you prescribed are running through.

B Come back in another 90 minutes as the nursing staff should, it is hoped, have the fluids set up by then.

C Fill out a critical incident form.

D Ask one of the nurses to put up the fluids for you now, explaining their importance in this case.

E Put up the fluids yourself even though you are not really sure how to set up an intravenous infusion.

5. You have started a new post and have noticed that the other senior house officer on the firm turns up for work late every day by at least 20 minutes, leaves every day 30 minutes before the end of shift and takes very long lunches.

   Which three of the following would you pick as your best course of action?

   A Inform her that you are likely to raise the matter to seniors if it keeps happening.

   B Take her aside somewhere quiet and private for an informal chat.

   C Do nothing as you have no time to talk to her.

   D Inform her that you are here to help in any way possible.

   E Sit down with other senior house officers at work and have an informal chat to see if they are aware of any problems your colleague may be going through currently.

6. You are seeing patients as part of your general practice rotation in surgery and see a patient previously seen by your educational supervisor. The patient advises you that at the previous appointment he was told he could have his travel claim form filled in at this appointment as he missed his holiday due to sickness. He also tells you he is in a hurry and needed to take time off work to come in and see you.

   Which three of the following would you pick as your best course of action?

   A Agree to fill in the form; it will not take long and the patient has already been advised that he can have the form.

   B Look through the notes for evidence of the last consultation to see if this was noted.

   C Ask the patient to wait while you step out to speak to your educational supervisor and find out what was discussed.

   D Refuse as you are in a hurry and this is not your role as GP.

   E Ask the patient to leave the paperwork with the reception staff who will forward it to the admin team for processing. Advise him there is a fee for this work.

7. You are on call for a busy medical team. You have been called to the Emergency Department to see a 79-year-old man who requires emergency resuscitation and you are currently working on a 22-year-old man on the ward with acute asthma.

Which of the three options would you choose as your next line of management?

A Call the Emergency Department and tell them to bleep your registrar and you will attend the Emergency Department as soon as your patient is stable.

B Ensuring your patient is stable, ask the charge nurse to observe the patient while you go to the Emergency Department. Ask another member of staff to page another member of the team.

C Call you registrar yourself and make sure he can come and help with one of the patients.

D Leave your patient and go to the Emergency Department.

E Ignore the bleep as you are busy; they should be able to find another member of the team.

8. You are seeing patients in a busy GP surgery during one of your GP rotations. Your educational supervisor walks into the room after your patient has left and advises you that he needs to go home to attend to some building work. You will be alone in the surgery. What three options would you choose as most appropriate?

A Lose your temper and storm out; you feel taken advantage of and have had a busy tiring morning already.

B Ask to discuss what will happen in the event of an emergency as you are alone and do not feel you would be adequately equipped to deal with an emergency.

C Take his mobile number and hope that nothing happens while he is not around; it is your first rotation with him and you do not wish to make waves.

D Ask if there are any other partners around that could supervise while he steps out.

E Express your discomfort at being left alone and discuss your role in the practice.

9. You are running 20 minutes late in your evening surgery and are the last person left in the building, apart from one reception staff member who is supervising the reception desk. You see a female patient who requires an intimate examination for a sexually transmitted infection. The patient is in a hurry and has already been kept waiting. Select three options for what you should do as the best course of action

A The patient is in a hurry so you will examine them this time without a chaperone.

B Make the diagnosis without examining them and hope you are right.

C Arrange for them to come on another day and they can be examined by you or someone else when a chaperone is present.

D Discuss the option of looking for a chaperone or rebooking an appointment and let the patient decide. Make it clear that you cannot examine and therefore diagnose her condition without a chaperone.

E Record the details of the consultation and ask her to rebook an appointment while giving her the local sexual health services number.

10. You are leaving the hospital to go home, and see a patient coming in who was admitted a few months earlier under your team. He does not speak any English and you spent a long time finding out his history and medical background which is complicated. Unfortunately he is not registered with a GP and so his history is difficult to access. The notes will not be available until the following day.

    What is the best course of action to take? Choose the three most suitable options.

    A Do not stop as you are exhausted and they will find his notes the next day anyway.
    B Call them as you are driving home and explain what you know.
    C Go back and see what has brought the patient in, explain the patient history to the treating team.
    D Write down as much information as you know in the temporary notes to ensure that the patient receives the best care possible.
    E Stay with the patient until they have been assessed to offer any help if needed.

Answers

Q1 C, D, B.

The main concern here is patient safety, as well as knowing your limitations. Options C and D involve appropriate patient management.

Option B is important as, despite it being late, you are concerned about a deterioration in the patient's state and hence family should be contacted if the patient is agreeable.

Option A is more suitable than option E as it involves admitting your deficiencies and informing the nursing staff that you are not experienced enough to handle such an unwell patient. Option E is problematic, to say the least. It disregards the unwell patient entirely and demonstrates a simple lack of patient care and professionalism.

Q2 D, C, E.

This issue is looking at the remit of communication skills, personal integrity and patient safety. The least appropriate action is option B, as this option ignores the problem entirely with the hope that it will resolve by itself. Contacting the GMC is the next least appropriate option, as it is only a minor error and you are not allowing your colleague a chance to be aware of your concern or address the error. The GMC should only be contacted as a last resort if the matter cannot be resolved locally.

Option E is the third least appropriate option as it is not dealing with the situation at that particular moment in time. Having said that, however, you are ensuring the prescribing errors are brought to the attention of the trust.

With regard to option C, it would be safe to say that as a junior doctor you will not feel well equipped to deal with such a matter alone and you may not feel entirely comfortable approaching your consultant directly, hence remaining vigilant is imperative.

Option D is the most appropriate option, bringing the error to light and asking for senior advice.

Q3 C, E, A.

Options F and G are completely inappropriate and a breach of patient confidentiality. Option D is the third least appropriate option as you are ignoring the family and their concerns. Option B is the next least appropriate option as you are not addressing the family's concerns, making them more likely to make a formal complaint against your colleagues, which implies poor professional integrity.

Options C, E and A are the most appropriate. They ensure that you will speak to the family and explain that you do not know the patient directly but that you will do your best to answer their questions. This shows that you are taking their concerns seriously and shows empathy for their situation.

Q4 D, A, C.

The least appropriate option is B as this is ignoring the situation completely and interfering with appropriate patient management.

Option D is the most suitable option as the patient is being managed immediately with appropriate fluid resuscitation.

Option E is the second least suitable option. Although you want to give the fluids intravenously as necessary, if you are unsure how to set up an infusion you are putting the patient at considerable risk.

You are then left with options A and C. Option A is the better of the two as you are ensuring the fluids will be running through. Option C is also important as it ensures the incident is being formally reported and can be looked into to prevent similar instances occurring in future.

Q5 B, D, A.

Option C is the least suitable option as it involves ignoring the situation at hand. Option B is the most preferred option as it involves questioning your colleague in a professional, dignified fashion. Option D also demonstrates your willingness to support her.

Option E, on the other hand, involves making your concerns public to other work colleagues which is not professional in the slightest. Option A is more suitable than option E as the matter is being raised to a senior colleague for further guidance if she continues to work in such a fashion.

Q6 B, C, E.

Options B, C and E are the most appropriate as in this case it would be prudent to find out exactly what was said at the last consultation (options B and C). If this was not possible it would be better to ask the patient to leave the paperwork (option E) and come back to collect it once completed, as this is the normal course for this type of work.

Option D, refusing a patient request outright, is unprofessional and inappropriate without discussion. Option A, agreeing to complete the form purely to pacify the patient, is also inappropriate, as part of working professionally involves appropriate use of time and resources.

Q7 A, B, C.

Options A, B and C show that you have prioritised patient care for both patients, but more importantly, your duty of care to the patient you are caring for is uncompromised.

The last two options are less responsible answers as option D neglects duty of care to the asthmatic patient and option E neglects the patient in the Emergency Department. Above all else, as a junior doctor in training, prioritisation of patient safety must always come first. Calling for help is always important as one of the first actions in any emergency patient care, as well as clear and effective communication.

Q8 B, D, E.

In this instance it would be very inappropriate for a foundation trainee to be left alone in a practice as there should be adequate educational supervision at all times. In addition, trainees should not be made to feel uncomfortable or unsafe in their practice as this will ultimately compromise patient safety.

It is, however, a difficult situation to be put in as it would require the trainee to take a stand and voice their discomfort. This is an important learning point as ultimately if an emergency did occur and patient care was compromised then the responsibility would still lie with the treating doctor for part of the outcome. Therefore it is important to always ensure adequate senior cover in all training posts and to voice concern if this is not the case.

Options A and C are less acceptable as they do not address the issue of senior supervision and leave the possibility of compromised patient care open.

Q9 C, D, E.

Options C, D and E all make it clear that you cannot complete an examination without a chaperone present in line with GMC guidance. They also give her options and offer a shared management plan. It is important to always ask a patient what their preferred choice is in how to proceed as, in this scenario, time and convenience may be more important for the patient and therefore she may be happy to go along to a sexual health clinic. However, for others the continuity of having her own doctor examine her may be more important and therefore she would rebook.

Options A and B offer poor patient care as they do not offer her any options and compromise patient care. Also, undertaking an intimate examination of the patient without a chaperone present could expose you, as a practitioner, to disciplinary action if the patient was unhappy or felt uncomfortable.

Q10 C, D, E.

Options C, D and E allow you to give the team treating the patient the most information and therefore the best chance of developing the most appropriate management plan. This is a question of probity and duty of care. It is important to always put a patient's interest first and this can sometimes conflict with a clinician's own needs. However in this instance the time taken to offer some extra clinical support would not require that much. It is however a more difficult dilemma when personal commitments become more pressurised.

In this scenario option B would be less reliable as the team may be busy or the patient may be very unwell and option A would neglect the duty altogether.

Index

The Complete GPVTS Stage 2 Preparation Guide: Questions and Professional Dilemmas, First Edition. Edited by Saba Khan with Neel Sharma.
© 2012 John Wiley & Sons, Ltd. Published 2012 by John Wiley & Sons, Ltd.